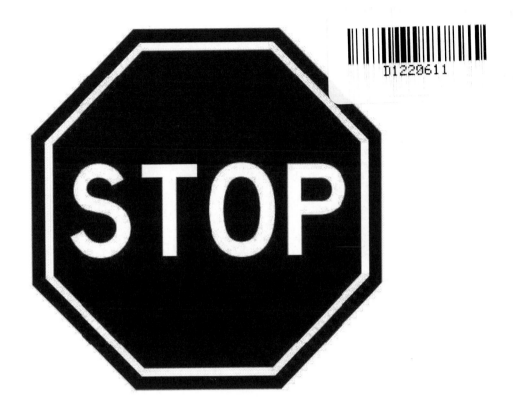

FREE Test Taking Tips DVD Offer

To help us better serve you, we have developed a Test Taking Tips DVD that we would like to give you for FREE. **This DVD covers world-class test taking tips that you can use to be even more successful when you are taking your test.**

All that we ask is that you email us your feedback about your study guide. Please let us know what you thought about it – whether that is good, bad or indifferent.

To get your **FREE Test Taking Tips DVD**, email freedvd@studyguideteam.com with "FREE DVD" in the subject line and the following information in the body of the email:

a. The title of your study guide.

b. Your product rating on a scale of 1-5, with 5 being the highest rating.

c. Your feedback about the study guide. What did you think of it?

d. Your full name and shipping address to send your free DVD.

If you have any questions or concerns, please don't hesitate to contact us at freedvd@studyguideteam.com.

Thanks again!

DTR Exam Study Guide

Dietetic Technician Registration Study Guide Team

Copyright © 2017 Dietetic Technician Registration Study Guide Team

All rights reserved.

Table of Contents

Quick Overview

As you draw closer to taking your exam, effective preparation becomes more and more important. Thankfully, you have this study guide to help you get ready. Use this guide to help keep your studying on track and refer to it often.

This study guide contains several key sections that will help you be successful on your exam. The guide contains tips for what you should do the night before and the day of the test. Also included are test-taking tips. Knowing the right information is not always enough. Many well-prepared test takers struggle with exams. These tips will help equip you to accurately read, assess, and answer test questions.

A large part of the guide is devoted to showing you what content to expect on the exam and to helping you better understand that content. Near the end of this guide is a practice test so that you can see how well you have grasped the content. Then, answer explanations are provided so that you can understand why you missed certain questions.

Don't try to cram the night before you take your exam. This is not a wise strategy for a few reasons. First, your retention of the information will be low. Your time would be better used by reviewing information you already know rather than trying to learn a lot of new information. Second, you will likely become stressed as you try to gain a large amount of knowledge in a short amount of time. Third, you will be depriving yourself of sleep. So be sure to go to bed at a reasonable time the night before. Being well-rested helps you focus and remain calm.

Be sure to eat a substantial breakfast the morning of the exam. If you are taking the exam in the afternoon, be sure to have a good lunch as well. Being hungry is distracting and can make it difficult to focus. You have hopefully spent lots of time preparing for the exam. Don't let an empty stomach get in the way of success!

When travelling to the testing center, leave earlier than needed. That way, you have a buffer in case you experience any delays. This will help you remain calm and will keep you from missing your appointment time at the testing center.

Be sure to pace yourself during the exam. Don't try to rush through the exam. There is no need to risk performing poorly on the exam just so you can leave the testing center early. Allow yourself to use all of the allotted time if needed.

Remain positive while taking the exam even if you feel like you are performing poorly. Thinking about the content you should have mastered will not help you perform better on the exam.

Once the exam is complete, take some time to relax. Even if you feel that you need to take the exam again, you will be well served by some down time before you begin studying again. It's often easier to convince yourself to study if you know that it will come with a reward!

Test-Taking Strategies

1. Predicting the Answer

When you feel confident in your preparation for a multiple-choice test, try predicting the answer before reading the answer choices. This is especially useful on questions that test objective factual knowledge or that ask you to fill in a blank. By predicting the answer before reading the available choices, you eliminate the possibility that you will be distracted or led astray by an incorrect answer choice. You will feel more confident in your selection if you read the question, predict the answer, and then find your prediction among the answer choices. After using this strategy, be sure to still read all of the answer choices carefully and completely. If you feel unprepared, you should not attempt to predict the answers. This would be a waste of time and an opportunity for your mind to wander in the wrong direction.

2. Reading the Whole Question

Too often, test takers scan a multiple-choice question, recognize a few familiar words, and immediately jump to the answer choices. Test authors are aware of this common impatience, and they will sometimes prey upon it. For instance, a test author might subtly turn the question into a negative, or he or she might redirect the focus of the question right at the end. The only way to avoid falling into these traps is to read the entirety of the question carefully before reading the answer choices.

3. Looking for Wrong Answers

Long and complicated multiple-choice questions can be intimidating. One way to simplify a difficult multiple-choice question is to eliminate all of the answer choices that are clearly wrong. In most sets of answers, there will be at least one selection that can be dismissed right away. If the test is administered on paper, the test taker could draw a line through it to indicate that it may be ignored; otherwise, the test taker will have to perform this operation mentally or on scratch paper. In either case, once the obviously incorrect answers have been eliminated, the remaining choices may be considered. Sometimes identifying the clearly wrong answers will give the test taker some information about the correct answer. For instance, if one of the remaining answer choices is a direct opposite of one of the eliminated answer choices, it may well be the correct answer. The opposite of obviously wrong is obviously right! Of course, this is not always the case. Some answers are obviously incorrect simply because they are irrelevant to the question being asked. Still, identifying and eliminating some incorrect answer choices is a good way to simplify a multiple-choice question.

4. Don't Overanalyze

Anxious test takers often overanalyze questions. When you are nervous, your brain will often run wild, causing you to make associations and discover clues that don't actually exist. If you feel that this may be a problem for you, do whatever you can to slow down during the test. Try taking a deep breath or counting to ten. As you read and consider the question, restrict yourself to the particular words used by the author. Avoid thought tangents about what the author *really* meant, or what he or she was *trying* to say. The only things that matter on a multiple-choice test are the words that are actually in the question. You must avoid reading too much into a multiple-choice question, or supposing that the writer meant something other than what he or she wrote.

5. No Need for Panic

It is wise to learn as many strategies as possible before taking a multiple-choice test, but it is likely that you will come across a few questions for which you simply don't know the answer. In this situation, avoid panicking. Because most multiple-choice tests include dozens of questions, the relative value of a single wrong answer is small. Moreover, your failure on one question has no effect on your success elsewhere on the test. As much as possible, you should compartmentalize each question on a multiple-choice test. In other words, you should not allow your feelings about one question to affect your success on the others. When you find a question that you either don't understand or don't know how to answer, just take a deep breath and do your best. Read the entire question slowly and carefully. Try rephrasing the question a couple of different ways. Then, read all of the answer choices carefully. After eliminating obviously wrong answers, make a selection and move on to the next question.

6. Confusing Answer Choices

When working on a difficult multiple-choice question, there may be a tendency to focus on the answer choices that are the easiest to understand. Many people, whether consciously or not, gravitate to the answer choices that require the least concentration, knowledge, and memory. This is a mistake. When you come across an answer choice that is confusing, you should give it extra attention. A question might be confusing because you do not know the subject matter to which it refers. If this is the case, don't eliminate the answer before you have affirmatively settled on another. When you come across an answer choice of this type, set it aside as you look at the remaining choices. If you can confidently assert that one of the other choices is correct, you can leave the confusing answer aside. Otherwise, you will need to take a moment to try to better understand the confusing answer choice. Rephrasing is one way to tease out the sense of a confusing answer choice.

7. Your First Instinct

Many people struggle with multiple-choice tests because they overthink the questions. If you have studied sufficiently for the test, you should be prepared to trust your first instinct once you have carefully and completely read the question and all of the answer choices. There is a great deal of research suggesting that the mind can come to the correct conclusion very quickly once it has obtained all of the relevant information. At times, it may seem to you as if your intuition is working faster even than your reasoning mind. This may in fact be true. The knowledge you obtain while studying may be retrieved from your subconscious before you have a chance to work out the associations that support it. Verify your instinct by working out the reasons that it should be trusted.

8. Key Words

Many test takers struggle with multiple-choice questions because they have poor reading comprehension skills. Quickly reading and understanding a multiple-choice question requires a mixture of skill and experience. To help with this, try jotting down a few key words and phrases on a piece of scrap paper. Doing this concentrates the process of reading and forces the mind to weigh the relative importance of the question's parts. In selecting words and phrases to write down, the test taker thinks about the question more deeply and carefully. This is especially true for multiple-choice questions that are preceded by a long prompt.

9. Subtle Negatives

One of the oldest tricks in the multiple-choice test writer's book is to subtly reverse the meaning of a question with a word like *not* or *except*. If you are not paying attention to each word in the question, you can easily be led astray by this trick. For instance, a common question format is, "Which of the following is...?" Obviously, if the question instead is, "Which of the following is not...?," then the answer will be quite different. Even worse, the test makers are aware of the potential for this mistake and will include one answer choice that would be correct if the question were not negated or reversed. A test taker who misses the reversal will find what he or she believes to be a correct answer and will be so confident that he or she will fail to reread the question and discover the original error. The only way to avoid this is to practice a wide variety of multiple-choice questions and to pay close attention to each and every word.

10. Reading Every Answer Choice

It may seem obvious, but you should always read every one of the answer choices! Too many test takers fall into the habit of scanning the question and assuming that they understand the question because they recognize a few key words. From there, they pick the first answer choice that answers the question they believe they have read. Test takers who read all of the answer choices might discover that one of the latter answer choices is actually *more* correct. Moreover, reading all of the answer choices can remind you of facts related to the question that can help you arrive at the correct answer. Sometimes, a misstatement or incorrect detail in one of the latter answer choices will trigger your memory of the subject and will enable you to find the right answer. Failing to read all of the answer choices is like not reading all of the items on a restaurant menu: you might miss out on the perfect choice.

11. Spot the Hedges

One of the keys to success on multiple-choice tests is paying close attention to every word. This is never more true than with words like *almost, most, some,* and *sometimes.* These words are called "hedges" because they indicate that a statement is not totally true or not true in every place and time. An absolute statement will contain no hedges, but in many subjects, like literature and history, the answers are not always straightforward or absolute. There are always exceptions to the rules in these subjects. For this reason, you should favor those multiple-choice questions that contain hedging language. The presence of qualifying words indicates that the author is taking special care with his or her words, which is certainly important when composing the right answer. After all, there are many ways to be wrong, but there is only one way to be right! For this reason, it is wise to avoid answers that are absolute when taking a multiple-choice test. An absolute answer is one that says things are either all one way or all another. They often include words like *every, always, best,* and *never.* If you are taking a multiple-choice test in a subject that doesn't lend itself to absolute answers, be on your guard if you see any of these words.

12. Long Answers

In many subject areas, the answers are not simple. As already mentioned, the right answer often requires hedges. Another common feature of the answers to a complex or subjective question are qualifying clauses, which are groups of words that subtly modify the meaning of the sentence. If the question or answer choice describes a rule to which there are exceptions or the subject matter is complicated, ambiguous, or confusing, the correct answer will require many words in order to be expressed clearly and accurately. In essence, you should not be deterred by answer choices that seem excessively long. Oftentimes, the author of the text will not be able to write the correct answer without offering some qualifications and modifications. Your job is to read the answer choices thoroughly and completely and to select the one that most accurately and precisely answers the question.

13. Restating to Understand

Sometimes, a question on a multiple-choice test is difficult not because of what it asks but because of how it is written. If this is the case, restate the question or answer choice in different words. This process serves a couple of important purposes. First, it forces you to concentrate on the core of the question. In order to rephrase the question accurately, you have to understand it well. Rephrasing the question will concentrate your mind on the key words and ideas. Second, it will present the information to your mind in a fresh way. This process may trigger your memory and render some useful scrap of information picked up while studying.

14. True Statements

Sometimes an answer choice will be true in itself, but it does not answer the question. This is one of the main reasons why it is essential to read the question carefully and completely before proceeding to the answer choices. Too often, test takers skip ahead to the answer choices and look for true statements. Having found one of these, they are content to select it without reference to the question above. Obviously, this provides an easy way for test makers to play tricks. The savvy test taker will always read the entire question before turning to the answer choices. Then, having settled on a correct answer choice, he or she will refer to the original question and ensure that the selected answer is relevant. The mistake of choosing a correct-but-irrelevant answer choice is especially common on questions related to specific pieces of objective knowledge, like historical or scientific facts. A prepared test taker will have a wealth of factual knowledge at his or her disposal, and should not be careless in its application.

15. No Patterns

One of the more dangerous ideas that circulates about multiple-choice tests is that the correct answers tend to fall into patterns. These erroneous ideas range from a belief that B and C are the most common right answers, to the idea that an unprepared test-taker should answer "A-B-A-C-A-D-A-B-A." It cannot be emphasized enough that pattern-seeking of this type is exactly the WRONG way to approach a multiple-choice test. To begin with, it is highly unlikely that the test maker will plot the correct answers according to some predetermined pattern. The questions are scrambled and delivered in a random order. Furthermore, even if the test maker was following a pattern in the assignation of correct answers, there is no reason why the test taker would know which pattern he or she was using. Any attempt to discern a pattern in the answer choices is a waste of time and a distraction from the real work of taking the test. A test taker would be much better served by extra preparation before the test than by reliance on a pattern in the answers.

FREE DVD OFFER

Don't forget that doing well on your exam includes both understanding the test content and understanding how to use what you know to do well on the test. We offer a completely FREE Test Taking Tips DVD that covers world class test taking tips that you can use to be even more successful when you are taking your test.

All that we ask is that you email us your feedback about your study guide. To get your **FREE Test Taking Tips DVD**, email freedvd@studyguideteam.com with "FREE DVD" in the subject line and the following information in the body of the email:

- The title of your study guide.
- Your product rating on a scale of 1-5, with 5 being the highest rating.
- Your feedback about the study guide. What did you think of it?
- Your full name and shipping address to send your free DVD.

Introduction to the DTR Exam

Function of the Test

The DTR (Dietetic Technician, Registered) exam, or Registration Exam for Dietetic Technicians is part of the Commission on Dietetic Registration's certification process. The exam is intended for those wishing to become certified dietary technicians as a means of demonstrating their education and training in dietetics practice and their understanding of providing safe and competent nutrition services and education to the public. Certified DTRs may work in schools, public health agencies, health clubs, or food vending and distributing corporations.

The DTR exam is available worldwide to those who meet the requirements detailed below, but most tests are administered in the United States or Canada. Typically, approximately two-thirds of test takers pass the exam, but the pass rate has fallen slightly in recent years. In 2012, the Council of Future Practice made a recommendation to discontinue the DTR credential entirely, but the Commission on Dietetic Registration (CDR) has said that it will continue to offer the DTR credential as long as it remains financially feasible for them to do so.

Test Administration

Individuals wishing to take the DTR exam must either 1) have completed at least an Associate's degree from an accredited U.S. college or foreign equivalent and have completed at least 450 supervised practice hours; or 2) have completed at least a baccalaureate degree from an accredited U.S. college or foreign equivalent and met certain academic requirements as outlined by the Accreditation Council for Education in Nutrition and Dietetics.

The CDR offers the DTR at over 250 Pearson VUE testing centers across the United States. Testing centers are typically open Monday through Friday, and sometimes on Saturdays. Test takers may schedule their exam for a day and time that is most convenient to them.

Test takers who do not pass the exam may retest any time, once 45 days have passed since their first attempt. Such test takers must be reauthorized as examination-eligible through the CDR and pay the current examination application fee. There is no limit on the number of retakes.

In accordance with the Americans With Disabilities Act, test takers with documented disabilities may receive appropriate accommodations.

Test Format

The DTR exam contains at least 110 questions and at most 130 questions and 30 of the included questions are unscored. All questions are multiple-choice. The exam lasts 2 hours and 30 minutes. The test taker must get through a minimum number of questions in the allotted time or the exam will not be scored.

The test varies in length because it is a computer-adaptive test. This means that the questions presented to a given test taker depend on his or her answers to previous questions. Depending on the test taker's performance, the questions may get easier or harder, or focus on different subject areas.

No electronic items or notes are allowed in the testing center. A simple "pop-up" calculator is available on-screen for use during the test.

Here's the breakdown of what the test covers:

Topic	Percentage of Test
Nutrition Science and Care for Individuals and Groups	44%
Food Science and Food Service	24%
Management of Food and Nutrition Services	32%

Scoring

The CDR determines the passing score by first surveying experienced dietetics professionals representing different practice areas to establish the minimum acceptable professional performance on the test material, A criterion-referenced approach is then used to determine the passing score, and to equate future exams to ensure various forms are of equivalent difficulty.

Scaled scores fall between 1 and 50, with a score of at least 25 required to pass. Test takers receive their score report upon completion of the exam. Score reports include the test taker's scaled score and the required scaled score to pass, as well as scaled scores on each subtopic within the exam.

Recent/Future Developments

Every five years, the CDR conducts an audit of the profession to update the content of the DTR exam. The most recent cycle concludes with an updated test (the content of which is described above) first offered in January 2017. Instead of the three subject categories covered by the new exam, the previous version covered five: 1) Food and Nutrition Sciences; 2) Nutrition Care for Individuals and Groups; 3) Principles, Education and Training; 4) Foodservice Systems; 5) Management of Food and Nutrition Services.

Nutrition Science and Care for Individuals and Groups

Principles of Basic and Normal Nutrition

Nutrients and Phytochemicals

Functions

Macronutrients are carbohydrates, fats, and protein that are important sources of energy for the body and are needed in large quantities. They contribute to the overall energy pool of the body.

Micronutrients are vitamins and minerals that function as coenzymes, co-catalysts, and buffers in metabolism.

Phytochemicals are naturally occurring substances found in plants that act as a natural defense system and have been shown to be beneficial to humans by reducing the risk for diseases such as cancer and cardiovascular disease.

Deficiencies and Excesses

Deficiencies in macronutrients or micronutrients can disrupt metabolism, exacerbate disease states, lower resistance to infection, and lead to poor wound healing. Some conditions, such as night blindness, are caused by a deficiency of vitamin A. Deficiencies in calcium and vitamin D can impair bone mineralization in children, causing rickets.

Excesses in macronutrients can lead to obesity and related conditions such as type 2 diabetes mellitus, cardiovascular disease, or metabolic syndrome. Certain micronutrients, such as Vitamin A, consumed in excess can cause toxicities, leading to liver damage.

Macronutrients Sources

Macronutrients are carbohydrates, proteins, and fats and are required in large amounts to support the human body:

- Carbohydrates: Contribute 4 kilocalories per gram.

  Food sources include fruits, vegetables, grains, starches, beans, breads. The most abundant sources of carbohydrates are starch, sugar, and fiber.

- Proteins: Contribute 4 kilocalories per gram.

  Food sources from animals typically provide all of the amino acids the human body needs (essential amino acids). Those sources include beef, poultry, fish, lamb, dairy products, and eggs. Non-animal sources of protein include beans, nuts, seeds, whole grains, some fruits and vegetables.

- Fats: Contribute 9 kilocalories per gram

  There are two main types of dietary fat: saturated and unsaturated. Most foods have a combination of saturated and unsaturated fats. Saturated fats are mainly found in animal sources (e.g. beef or cheese) but can also be found in coconut, coconut oil, palm oil, and palm kernel oil. Saturated fats have no available sites for hydrogen atoms to bond, so they are solid at room temperature and have a longer shelf life than unsaturated fats.

The two types of unsaturated fats are monounsaturated and polyunsaturated and they are found in the highest concentrations in plant-based foods. Unsaturated fatty acids still have available sites for hydrogen to bond (monounsaturated fats like in olives, avocados, canola and peanut oil have one double-bonded carbon, while polyunsaturated fats have multiple double-bonds like in corn, safflower, and sesame oils), so they are less stable and liquid (oil) at room temperature.

Olive, peanut and canola oils, avocado, nuts, and seeds contain high levels of monounsaturated fats. Sunflower, corn, soybean and flaxseed oils, walnuts, flax seeds, and fish have high concentrations of polyunsaturated fats. Note that although canola oil consists of mostly monounsaturated fats (approximately (61%), it also has 32% polyunsaturated fats (with the remainder as saturated fats). Therefore, it is considered a good source of both types of unsaturated fats.

Omega-3 fatty acids are important polyunsaturated fats and must come from dietary sources. Good sources of these fatty acids include fish, ground flaxseeds, walnuts, canola oil, and soybean oil.

Hydrogenation is a process that converts unsaturated fatty acids to saturated fatty acids, which changes the structure of the fatty acid. It contributes to the stability and shelf life of products such as chips, crackers, frosting, candy, and pastry. Fat that has been hydrogenated stays solid at room temperature and prevents the oil in the product from weeping. Trans fatty acids are synthetically made and have been scientifically shown to increase the risk of heart disease.

Micronutrients Sources
Micronutrients are vitamins and minerals needed only in small quantities. They must be obtained from the diet to support a healthy immune system, tissue repair, growth and development in children, and overall health and wellbeing.

Micronutrients are available in a wide variety of food sources including fruits, vegetables, grains, beef, poultry, and dairy products. Fortification of certain products such as breads and breakfast cereals have become an important source of some micronutrients (such as folate) in the typical American diet. A few important micronutrients include iron, zinc, vitamin A, folate, zinc, calcium, and vitamin D.

Basic Human Physiology, Physical, and Biological Sciences

Ingestion
In humans, ingestion is the act of consuming a food or beverage usually through the mouth and into the gastrointestinal tract.

(duodenum → jejunum → ileum)

Digestion   mouth → esophagus → stomach → SI → LI
Digestion begins in the mouth during the process of chewing food, continues in the stomach, and concludes in the small intestine. Digestion is an important physiological process, breaking down macro- and micro- nutrients into smaller, more easily absorbed forms that can be utilized by the body. Food is moved through the esophagus and intestine via peristalsis. Peristalsis is a series of coordinated muscle movements that constrict and relax or squeeze and shorten to propel the food. Digestion and absorption of most of the food and beverages ingested takes place in the first 100cm of the small intestine. Most digestion is complete by the middle of the jejunum.

The upper and lower esophageal sphincters are responsible for how food flows through the esophagus. The lower esophageal sphincter stops food from moving back from the stomach into the esophagus and causing heartburn or reflux related symptoms. Age, weight status, and diet can interfere with the function of the lower esophageal sphincter, causing uncomfortable symptoms that may have to be managed with medication or diet modification.

The food matrix influences the rate of stomach emptying. Foods rich in protein and carbohydrates empty from the stomach at about the same rate. Complex carbohydrates and high fat foods take longer to digest. Gastric emptying following a meal typically requires between two and six hours.

Digestion is regulated by several hormones:

- Cholecystokinin (CCK): secreted by the proximal small bowel and stimulates the pancreas to secrete enzymes, slows gastric emptying, stimulates gallbladder contraction and colonic activity, and may regulate appetite.

- Secretin: released from the duodenal wall and stimulates the pancreas to secrete water and bicarbonate. It inhibits gastric acid secretion and stomach emptying. Secretin is stimulated by the presence of food in the stomach and the smell or sight of food. Wine, caffeine, food extracts, or partially digested proteins can stimulate secretin production and release.

- Gastrin: produced in the stomach and stimulates gastric secretions and motility.

Absorption

The small intestine is the primary location of nutrient and water absorption. The small intestine has an enormous absorptive area due to its length, folds, and brush border. A healthy individual with a fully functional small intestine has the capability to absorb far more calories and nutrients than needed to maintain optimum physiologic status.

Absorption is a complex process that is accomplished via passive diffusion or active transport.

- Passive diffusion: the movement of particles through openings in the cellular membranes according to electrochemical and concentration gradients.

- Facilitated diffusion: utilizes a transporter or carrier protein to move particles across a membrane.

- Active transport: requires the input of energy and the use of a carrier protein to move particles across cell members and epithelial layers. Active transport moves particles against the concentration gradient.

- Pinocytosis: allows large particles to be absorbed in small quantities. An example of pinocytosis is the absorption of the immunoglobulins in breast milk.

Blood sugar is controlled by several hormones:

- Insulin: made in the Beta cells of the pancreas and increases cell permeability to glucose.

- Glucagon: made in the Alpha cells of the pancreas and encourages the breakdown of glycogen to produce glucose (glycogenolysis)

- Glucocorticoids: encourage the breakdown of proteins to produce glucose (gluconeogenesis)

- Epinephrine: encourages the release of liver and muscle stores of glycogen to produce glucose (glycogenolysis) and decreases the release of insulin from the pancreas. Blood sugar increases during catabolic stress.

Growth hormones are insulin antagonists.

Insulin is responsible for lowering blood sugar while all other hormones raise blood sugar levels.

Metabolism/Utilization

The metabolic rate in the human body is affected by several variables including body size and composition, age, gender, and hormonal status. External factors such as the intake of caffeine, nicotine, and alcohol use also influence metabolic rate.

BMR

The basal metabolic rate is the minimal energy expenditure necessary to maintain body temperature, heartbeat, breathing, and other essential functions to keep the body alive. The amount of lean muscle mass is a primary factor in determining an individual's basal metabolic rate.

Carbohydrates are broken down into simple sugars, beginning in the mouth, but primarily in the intestines. In the liver, the simple sugars are converted to glucose for immediate use or glycogen for storage. Glucose is the only fuel utilized by the brain. Glucose is oxidized in cells to produce energy, carbon dioxide, and water.

Proteins are broken down into amino acids and sent to the tissues via the portal bloodstream. Proteins are oxidized to produce carbon dioxide and water, which releases heat and energy. Amino acids are not stored by the body.

Fats are broken down into monoglycerides, diglycerides, glycerol, and fatty acids. Fat metabolism requires an adequate supply of carbohydrates for complete oxidation. End products of fat digestion can be used as fuel or stored in adipose tissue or the liver. The liver is the primary location of lipid metabolism and is responsible for the production of triglycerides, makes cholesterol from triglycerides, de-saturate fatty acids, and breaks down triglycerides to use as an energy source.

Excretion

Excretion is necessary for the human body to eliminate waste products from metabolism. The major organs involved in excretion are the skin, lungs, kidneys, liver, large intestine, and gall bladder. The skin plays a small role in excretion by producing perspiration of which the main goal is to control body temperature. In humans, the lungs allow for exhalation of carbon dioxide from the blood stream to maintain the proper pH. The kidneys remove urea, salts, and excess water. The liver breaks down chemicals or other toxins that enter the body. The large intestine collects waste from the entire body and transports food particles to be expelled. The gallbladder stores and concentrates the bile, which is produced by the liver. Bile is secreted into the small intestine from bile ducts in the gallbladder in response to fats in the digestive tract. Bile helps emulsify fats, breaking the large fatty molecules into smaller ones with greater surface area. In this way, bile plays a crucial role in the digestion and absorption of fats. It also contributes to alkalizing the chyme as it moves from the acidic stomach environment into the intestines.

Body Systems

- Gastrointestinal system (GI): begins at the mouth and concludes at the anus. Responsible for digestion, absorption of nutrients, elimination of waste products.

- Cardiovascular system: composed of the heart and blood vessels. Responsible for circulating blood and oxygen through the body.

- Musculoskeletal system: composed of bones, cartilage, ligaments, and muscles. Bones protect internal organs, serve as attachment points for muscles, produce blood cells, and store calcium and phosphorus.

- Respiratory system: composed of the lungs and other organs that are responsible for taking in oxygen and expelling carbon dioxide.

- Endocrine system: composed of glands that produce hormones that regulate growth, metabolism, reproduction, sleep, sexual function, and tissue function.

- Renal system: composed of the kidneys, ureters, and bladder. Responsible for the production, storage, and elimination of urine.

- Immune system: composed of the lymph nodes and specialized cells that are designed to protect the body against harmful bacteria, viruses, and free radicals.

- Integumentary system: composed of skin, hair, nails, and sweat glands. It serves as the first line of defense against the environment and potentially harmful bacteria and viruses. Skin, hair, and nails are largely protective while the sweat glands help regulate body temperature and excrete wastes.

Nutrient and Calorie Needs at Various Stages of the Life Span

Dietary Reference Intakes (DRI) replaced the Recommended Dietary Allowances (RDA) and should be used to help people determine the adequacy of their diet. The DRI was designed to be more specific than the RDA by breaking down nutrient recommendations into three categories: estimated average requirement (EAR), adequate intake (AI), and tolerable upper intake levels (UL). The EAR provides nutrient recommendations that meet the needs of 50 percent of the population. An AI statement is issued if not enough data exists to make specific recommendations about a substance. It is assumed that this value is sufficient in healthy individuals. It is important to pay attention to UL levels and consumption about the recommendations could lead to potential toxicity.

Energy, protein, and nutrient recommendations determined by the DRI are based on metabolically normal children with normal body composition, activity, and growth. The DRIs may not be applicable in specific disease states or conditions (such as Down's Syndrome or Cystic Fibrosis). Critically ill, severely injured, or malnourished adults and children will also have different energy, protein, and micronutrient needs.

Infancy

Breast milk is the ideal food for infants. When this is not possible or is contraindicated, the use of iron-fortified infant formula is the best substitute. Breast milk and infant formula have approximately 20 calories per ounce. Infant formulas have more protein and iron than human milk but lack the antibodies found in human breast milk. The antibodies are important to the development of the infant immune system.

Complimentary foods should be introduced between four and six months of age when the baby is developmentally ready. Developmental cues that baby is ready for complimentary foods include the ability to hold up the head, the ability to sit up for longer periods of time, and the ability to pull the tongue back into the mouth. Families may choose to seek the opinion of an allergist prior to starting solid foods if there is a family history of food allergies.

Full-term infants should regain their birth weight between day ten and day fourteen of life. They should double their birth weight between five and six months of age and it should triple by the time the child is twelve months old.

Any infant that experiences a growth change of greater than two major percentiles (up or down) should be further evaluated.

Infants are classified based on their weight. An extremely low birth weight infant weighs less than 1,000 grams, and a low birth weight infant weighs less than 2,500 grams. Normal birth weight is considered between 2,500 and 4,000 grams.

Of all life stages, infancy requires the most calories, fat, protein, and water per gram of body weight. Between birth and six months, a normally developing infant requires approximately 550 calories per day, 9.1 grams of protein, and a minimum of 30 grams of fat per day. Fluid needs are based on age and range between 125 and 155 mL per kilogram of body weight. Between six and twelve months, normally developing infants require approximately 700 calories per day, 13.5 grams of protein, still require a minimum of 30 grams of fat daily. Fluid needs can be calculated at 1.5 mL per calorie or based on body weight.

Babies will need additional iron in the diet starting at around three months of age when fetal iron stores diminish. Families using bottled water or well water to mix infant formula should provide a fluoride supplement after six months of age. Exclusively breast fed babies should be given a vitamin D supplement.

Cow's milk should not be provided for the first twelve months of life. Low fat and non-fat milks should not be provided for the first two years of life due to the high need for fat in the diet.

Childhood
Starting around two years of age, children can gain an average of 4.5 to 6.5 pounds per year and can grow between 2.5 and 3.5 inches per year. Between one and three years of age, growth rate slows. Between four and six years of age, growth occurs in spurts and slows again between seven and ten years of age. The final growth spurt occurs during adolescence. Growth rates can vary greatly in children.

Trends in growth should be assessed regularly and children should follow their curve on the growth chart. As in infancy, any child that experiences a growth change of greater than two major percentiles (up or down) should be further evaluated.

Failure to thrive in childhood may be due to acute or chronic illness, a very restricted diet, poor diet choices, or chronic constipation that can lead to a decreased appetite.

Children should be proportional on their growth charts; for example, a child who is measured on the 75th percentile for height, should be on or near the 75th percentile for weight.

BMI is measured and used as a tool to determine if the child is considered to be at a healthy weight. It should be used with caution as human error in measurements can lead to misinterpretation of growth. Tall children will often have a higher BMI and may not be overweight or obese. A child is considered underweight with a BMI under the 5th percentile, a healthy weight if between the 5th and 84th percentile, overweight between the 84th and 94th percentile, and obese above the 95th percentile.

Adolescence
Adolescents experience rapid growth until puberty. The use of Tanner Staging can help determine how the child is progressing through adolescence.

Girls may begin their growth spurt as early as nine to ten years of age and can grow an average of 3 to 3.5 inches per year. Boys can begin their growth spurt around ten-and-a-half to eleven years of age and can grow and average of 3.5 to 4 inches per year. Growth velocity decreases once the adolescent reaches puberty. When assessing a child's growth history, take the parents' height into consideration. As in childhood, any adolescent that experiences a growth change of greater than two major percentiles (up or down) should be further evaluated. Calorie, protein, and fat requirements change in different disease states or conditions.

Adulthood CHO 45-65%. FAT 20-35%. PRO 10-35%.

Metabolism is influenced by any disease states, conditions, hormonal status, body composition, and physical activity. For a healthy adult, carbohydrates should comprise approximately 45 percent to 65 percent of total caloric intake, fat should make up approximately 20 percent to 35 percent of total caloric intake, while protein should make up the balance; approximately 10 percent to 35 percent. Target cholesterol intake should be less than 300 mg per day. Food labels and eating patterns such as MyPlate are based on a 2,000 calorie diet. This may not be an appropriate eating pattern for all adults, based on metabolism and physical activity levels. The MyPlate eating pattern does include an allowance for discretionary calories that come from added sugars, fats, oils, and alcohol. The goal in this dietary plan is no more than 265 discretionary calories daily.

The typical American diet is low in fiber. Current guidelines recommend that men under the age of fifty should consume at least 38 grams daily and women should consume 25 grams daily. The recommendations are lowered to 30 grams in men and 21 grams in women if over fifty years of age. It is important that anyone increasing fiber in their diet also has adequate fluid intake. Increasing fiber without increasing fluid could cause constipation.   (0.8 g/kg = protein needs)

The RDA for protein intake for healthy adults over nineteen years of age is approximately 56 grams in males and 46 grams in females. Certain disease states, such as cancer, or conditions such as wounds, require an increased protein intake. Adequate fluid intake is important in diets that are higher in protein to assist with kidney clearance.

Woman are encouraged to limit alcohol consumption to one drink per day while men should limit alcohol consumption to no more than two drinks per day.

Fluid intake in healthy adults is typically calculated at 1 mL per calorie or 35 mL per kilogram body weight.

Water is important during physical activity. Fluid, carbohydrate, and sodium are needed during and after exercise to maintain and restore hydration status.

Physical activity should be encouraged in all adults that are able to safely participate. Current recommendations state thirty minutes of moderate intensity activity is encouraged most days of the week to reduce the risk of chronic disease and sixty minutes of moderate-vigorous intensity activity most days of the week is recommended to help manage weight and promote gradual weight loss. To sustain weight loss, sixty to ninety minutes of moderate intensity physical activity most days of the week is recommended with an appropriate caloric intake.

It is important to ask patients about supplement use, including multivitamin/mineral supplements, powders, herbals, and botanicals. Supplement labels may contain structure/function claims but cannot make any claims about curing or treating specific conditions or diseases.

Certain botanicals can interfere with medications or cause organ dysfunction. Examples include ginkgo biloba and garlic supplements, which may change clotting time and interfere with warfarin. Black cohosh may cause blood clotting. Valerian root should not be used in individuals with liver disease.

Pregnancy and Lactation

Weight gain guidelines during pregnancy are based on the woman's pre-pregnant BMI. The goal is to achieve at least the lower limit in the range. Research indicates that women who gain excessive weight during pregnancy have a more difficult time returning to their pre-pregnancy weight. Very young women are encouraged to gain at the upper end of the guidelines to reduce the risk of complications. The weight gain pattern for a woman with a BMI in the normal weight range should be about one pound per week starting with the second trimester.

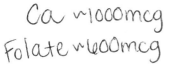

Pre-Pregnancy BMI	Weight Gain Guidelines
19.8 – 25.9	25 – 35 pounds
Under 19.8	28 – 40 pounds
26.0 – 29	15 – 25 pounds
Greater than 29	11 – 20 pounds

To meet the weight gain recommendations, a woman does not need to increase her caloric intake during the first trimester to meet fetal demands. Calorie needs increase by approximately 340 calories during the second trimester and 452 calories by the third, to meet the demands of the growing fetus.

During lactation, a woman can use fat stores accumulated during pregnancy to help achieve the caloric demands. In general, lactation places a demand of an additional 330 calories per day during the first six months and approximately 400 additional calories per day starting with month six. Breastfeeding women should be encouraged to maintain a healthy diet and not actively seek additional calories, unless they are experiencing rapid, unintentional weight loss or a decrease in their milk supply.

Women who fail to gain at least four pounds per month during the second half of pregnancy, are under the age of fifteen, over the age of thirty-five, or have had less than twelve months between pregnancies are considered at an increased risk for pregnancy-related complications.

All pregnant and lactating women should take a prenatal multivitamin/mineral supplement to help meet the demands of the fetus. Prenatal vitamins provide a greater amount of needed micronutrients than a standard multivitamin/mineral supplement. An iron supplement may be needed during the second and third trimester. Iron supplements should be taken between meals and not with milk, tea, or coffee, which can hinder absorption. The food matrix of a meal, including the calcium content, can interfere with iron absorption, and vitamin C can aid absorption. Pregnant women should get about 600 mcg of folate daily to reduce risk of neural tube defects. Women under the age of eighteen need about 1,300 mcg of calcium while women over the age of eighteen need about 1,000 mcg during pregnancy and lactation.

DHA, an omega 3 fatty acid, is important in the development of the fetal nervous system. It is added to prenatal vitamin supplements and infant formula to help meet fetal and infant demands.

Geriatric

One in five adults will be over the age of sixty-five by 2030, so this is a rapidly growing segment of the American population. Older adults are often willing to make dietary changes if it helps them maintain their independence and quality of life. Dietary advice should be sensitive to any chronic conditions and any mobility limitations.

Aging brings about changes in body composition. Fat mass and visceral fat increase while lean muscle mass decreases (sarcopenia). This can impact a person's ability to safely engage in physical activity. Metabolic rates also change in response to changes in body composition. Weight-bearing activity can slow the rate of these body changes.

Energy needs decline by approximately 3 percent per decade. Low calorie diets may be deficient in essential nutrients, so it is prudent to encourage older adults to seek nutrient-dense foods that provide sufficient amounts of micronutrients. Depending on the regular diet, supplements of folate and vitamins D, B6, and B12 may be needed depending on dietary intake.

Protein needs usually do not change with aging in a normal, healthy adult. Certain disease states or conditions such as wound healing may increase protein requirements. Kidney function may decline with age, so excess protein could be putting additional stress on the kidneys.

Older adults may suffer from constipation more often due to decreased gastric motility and reduced secretion of hydrochloric acid in the stomach. This can decrease appetite and cause unintentional weight loss. Adequate fluid intake can also help ease constipation. Recommendations are a minimum of 1,500 mL per day or 30 to 35 mL per kilogram body weight. Dehydration in older adults may present as confusion, falls, weakness, change in functional status, or fatigue and may go undiagnosed. Older adults may self restrict fluid intake due to fears of incontinence or decreased mobility.

An older adult should seek the advice of a health care professional before beginning exercise routines or dietary changes to promote weight loss. However, participation in regular physical activity should be encouraged to slow the age-related declines.

Encourage older adults to follow all food safety guidelines, as that population may be more susceptible to food poisoning and food borne illness.

Cultural Awareness

With the goal of providing clients with the most effective and successful health and nutrition treatment programming, nutrition professionals must consider several factors that can affect the development of a client's unique treatment plan. Religion, ethnicity, gender, and race are among those factors that can have a profound influence on an individual's lifestyle, diet, and health, as well as impact the components and approach to nutritional guidance and programming. To create an effective treatment plan, respect and appreciation for these aspects of one's identity must be prioritized. The likelihood of successful implementation of the information, advice, and instruction pertaining to the client's suggested program provided by the nutrition professional is increased if these factors are integrated throughout the entire process of the nutritional counseling and program design personalized for each client.

Religion
There are a variety of religions and faiths commonplace today, so it is imperative that a registered dietetic technician understand the nutritional and dietary guidelines practiced in various religions. The nutritional restrictions and practices of specific religions may require tailoring specific programs to permit adherence. For example, some individuals who observe Ramadan fast during daylight hours over this period; therefore, programs must be sensitive to this nutrient timing. Those following Kosher practices set forth by sects of Judaism may adhere to restrictions regarding the preparation practices of foods and meats, acceptable cuts of meat, food combinations, and foods to avoid altogether (such as pork and shellfish). Many Hindus do not consume beef, as the cow is sacred, and may follow lacto-vegetarian diets. Rastafarians typically avoid meat, seafood, and canned goods. Individuals practicing Jainism may consume diets devoid of meat, poultry, eggs, dairy, fish, and even root vegetables. Because these types of restrictions interfere with nutritional programming, a client's religion and the associated restrictions should be discussed and considered prior to the program's design.

Ethnicity

A client's ethnic identity can influence the nutritional staples, food preparation methods, and preferences in his or her diet. These factors should be identified and discussed during an intake appointment and addressed in the personalized programming for that client. A client's cultural or ethnic identity may prioritize or incorporate specific dishes, foods, or spices in his or her normal fare; for example, individuals from India may be accustomed to curries and lentil stews. Eskimos and Inuits may be used to fatty fish and sea mammals and somewhat unaccustomed to fresh fruits and vegetables. Dietetic technicians should take care to include culturally inclined foods in order to promote comfort and adherence to the proposed program. However, it should be noted that this information should be garnered during the interview and intake process rather than assumed, to avoid stereotyping, and potentially offending, clients.

Gender Sensitivity

Men and women require different nutritional recommendations unique to their differing body compositions, metabolic rates, hormonal profiles, and requirements for basic functioning. As a function of body size and composition, women tend to need fewer calories, more iron and calcium, and less protein than men, although this is a gross generalization and each client must be uniquely considered. Nutrition professionals should also consider motivation, societal pressures and expectations, and "ideal" body image for each gender and tailor counseling approaches to the varying needs of clients. For example, although these are stereotypes, it is true that some men can feel social pressure to consume "manly" foods (such as steak over salad) in the presence of others and some women may feel social or media pressure to conform to typical dieting practice of females, such as skipping meals or consuming "diet foods."

Race

Racial identity can impact the communication techniques that are most effective when working with a client. Nutrition professionals should always be sensitive to and respectful of racial identity when communicating with clients, both verbally and while presenting written questionnaires. An environment that celebrates diversity and acceptance should be fostered. It is important that nutrition professionals are mindful to not make assumptions about a client's racial identity simply from his or her appearance, but wait for the client to choose to self-disclose such information.

Nutrition Requirements in Health Promotion and Disease Prevention

As mentioned, nutrition requirements for health promotion and disease prevention vary throughout the lifecycle with changes in body size and composition, growth and development, and activity level. Effective programming must consider a client's age and life stage in addition to any pertinent medical information and/or special needs.

Infancy

During infancy, it is essential that a child remains adequately nourished for proper growth and development. While the saying "breast is best" embraces the ideal nutrition being provided to the infant by the mother, there are possibilities of malnourishment and deficiencies that can still occur with breast milk, particularly if maternal nutrition is poor. Additionally, after six months of age, infants can be susceptible to micronutrients, such as iron, if breast milk is not supplemented with nutrient-dense weaning foods, even if nursing from healthy mothers. In times of need, liquid vitamin and mineral supplements and fortified formulas can be integrated into infants' diet to ensure all nutritional needs are met. Infants should be monitored for adequate growth and weight gain. An infant's pediatrician or specialist should always be consulted when addressing areas of need for health and nutrition programming.

Infants that are formula-fed should be monitored for adequate growth and development. The specific formula of choice may be best selected after trying several and assessing which is best tolerated. Various protein sources are used in different formulas that may agree with the infant to varying degrees of success. Many infants that are formula fed grow more rapidly and gain weight faster than breastfed babies. If this becomes a concern, overfeeding should be addressed so that weight gain is not unhealthy.

Childhood

In toddlers and children, nutritional requirements may vary widely according to age, sex, activity level, and genetic predisposition to illness and disease. Regardless as to the specific caloric or nutrient needs, the focus across the board should be nutrient-dense foods in a balanced diet of protein, carbohydrates, and healthy fats. There should be an emphasis on including a variety of fruits, vegetables, eggs, nuts, seeds, dairy, and whole grains, with the main goal of providing essential macronutrients and micronutrients from whole, natural foods. Calcium and phosphorus are critical for healthy bone development. The registered dietetic technician should also make a point to explain that a child's exposure to a variety of healthy foods has shown to improve their chances of making healthy food choices throughout life as they age. Children should eat small, frequent meals and snacks every couple of hours throughout the day, and the importance of breakfast cannot be overstated. School breakfast, lunch, and milk programs, as well as summer supplemental programs, should be used for those with financial restrictions or income qualification. As with infants, a child's pediatrician or specialist should always be consulted when addressing areas of concern related to health and/or nutrition programming.

Adolescence

Adolescent clients' nutritional needs are affected by age, size, gender, BMI, activity level, and medical history. As growth usually occurs in spurts and is hormone-driven, nutrient needs are likely to change frequently in accordance with development and growth rate. Generally speaking, 60 to 80 kcal/kg is recommended to support periods of rapid growth. As girls begin menstruation, iron needs increase. Calcium and phosphorus, like in childhood, are crucial for healthy bone development. Clients in this age range are often most susceptible to eating disorders and unhealthy dieting practices. However, obesity is also a growing concern in this age group, especially in those who consume non-dairy sweetened beverages regularly.

Adulthood

As with adolescent clients, adult clients require in-depth assessments in order to provide the safest and most effective nutrition programs unique to each individual. With in-depth assessments, interviews, examinations, or questionnaires, the registered dietetic technician can provide a specialized nutrition program that helps the client reach their specific health goals in the safest and most effective manner. All clients should be encouraged to consume a healthy, varied diet, rich in whole foods, vegetables, fruits, proteins, legumes, and whole grains. Refined and processed food, sweetened beverages, and artificial sweeteners should be limited as much as possible.

Pregnancy and Lactation

Pregnant clients require specialized nutrition programming that takes into account a variety of factors including the client's trimester, health goals, food aversions and preferences, lifestyle habits, and medical history. Illnesses and health conditions unique to pregnancy, such as gestational diabetes and preeclampsia, require special nutritive care. Ideally, the registered dietetic technician should consider the pregnant client's current stage of pregnancy, risk factors and overall health, avoidance of potentially harmful foods such as certain fish and raw, unpasteurized dairy products, and the client's medical recommendations from their attending obstetrician. Proper nutrition is crucial for the developing fetus and pregnant women. Pregnant women who are insufficiently nourished are at increased risk of premature birth and/or having infants with compromised growth and development. Generally speaking, pregnant women require an additional 300 kcal per day and lactating women need 500 kcal a day over normal requirements. During pregnancy, growth of fetal tissues, the placenta, amniotic fluid, and blood volume create the need for an additional 10 grams of protein per day. Prenatal vitamins with folic acid should be encouraged prior to conceiving, to prevent spina bifida; in many cases, these supplements are helpful throughout pregnancy.

Geriatric

With a higher prevalence of illness and disease, the geriatric patient requires a more in-depth assessment to ensure that the recommended nutrition program adheres to the primary care physician's recommendations, avoids or eliminates potentially harmful foods, and includes natural foods that provide essential macronutrients and micronutrients. With cardiovascular, respiratory, muscular, and skeletal issues becoming more prevalent with advancing age, a focus on daily consumption of whole fruits, vegetables, grains, and healthy fats that provide an abundance of essential vitamins and minerals should be central in any nutrition program.

There are several factors unique to the aging population that should be considered when developing nutrition plans. Senses, especially taste and smell, can become less acute, which can reduce the extent to which geriatric adults taste sweet and salty foods. Consequently, they may compensate by adding an increased amount of salt or sugar to foods, which can be unhealthy. With aging, the gastric environment becomes more basic, and this reduction in gastric acidity (along with the frequent reliance on antacids in this population) can interfere with the absorption of vitamin B12, which is especially problematic in vegan individuals. Nutrition professionals should encourage supplementation when necessary and consult with medical providers with concerns for thalassemia. With changes in lifestyle habits, many older adults spend less time outdoors. Coupled with changes in the skin, this can impair vitamin D synthesis and absorption, so supplementation may need to be considered. Postmenopausal women should especially be encouraged to increase vitamin D and calcium intake. The thirst mechanism is thought to decrease with advancing age, so fluid intake should be stressed, and fluid balance should be monitored in some cases. Lastly, caloric needs decrease with lowering levels of activity and age-related changes in body composition, characterized as declining skeletal muscle mass (sarcopenia).

Screening and Assessment

Nutrition Screening

Nutrition screening and assessment is a crucial component of successful nutrition guidance, meal planning, and disease management. It involves the systematic, comprehensive process of gathering, verifying, and analyzing a patient's nutrition-related data. The process involves obtaining data related to dietary intake, psychosocial and behavioral factors related to diet, knowledge and readiness for change, and nutrition-related consequences of current health conditions. The data is compared to relevant standards and recommendations. Finally, possible problem areas are identified so that workable solutions can be addressed.

Purpose

The purpose of conducting thorough nutrition screening and assessment is to obtain complete data that can be analyzed and interpreted to best understand the baseline or current nutrition-related conditions and needs of clients. Nutritional issues can be a root or contributing cause of many physical, emotional, and even dental health issues. Without adequate and systematic screening, deficiencies, excesses, and other dietary problems can be overlooked. Nutrition-related issues can also influence acute and chronic disease conditions.

Selection and Use of Risk Factors

Data obtained from dietary assessments and screenings can yield information about nutrition risk factors for patients. Identification of such risk factors may indicate the need for further assessment or counseling. The following are indicators of possible nutrition risks in patients:

- Patients who report consuming fewer than three servings of vegetables per day
- Patients who report consuming fewer than two servings of fruit per day
- Patients who consume fewer than two servings of dairy daily or have a dairy intolerance   *Food choices*
- Patients who consume more than 20 oz. of soft drinks, excessive sugar and fat intake
- Patients who consume fewer than two servings of protein
- Patients with an unhealthy BMI
- Patients with diagnosed or a family history of cardiovascular or metabolic diseases

In addition to issues with food choices, issues with food resources can also increase risk. For example, patients lacking the financial resources to buy healthy food and those without access to food, nutrition education, or cooking facilities may be unable to provide themselves or their families with adequate nutrition. Eating behaviors that increase nutrition risk include the following:

- Patients with poor appetites, chronic diseases, depression, stress, or eating disorders
- Patients who frequent fast-food establishments more than three times per week
- Patients who skip meals several times per week
- Patients with hypercholesteremia or hyperlipedemia – *High cholesteral/Lipids*
- Patients with Amenorrhea or anemia – *lack of periods / Lack of RBC*
- Patients with digestive disorders like celiac disease

Additional indicators of nutrition risks include excessive or inadequate physical activity, those who have experienced significant weight changes in the prior six months, stunted growth in children and adolescents, and those with excessive concern about body shape or size, chronic dieting, purging, or use of laxatives. Further screening may be necessary for clients who use nutritional supplements, take prescribed medications, are pregnant, homeless, consume excessive alcohol or tobacco, and those with physical disabilities limiting the ability to feed themselves.

Values and Limitations

Experienced and educated nutrition professionals have a variety of assessment tools and protocols available for use with clients. Selecting the most appropriate assessment or battery of tests requires weighing the benefits and limitations of each screening tool within the context of the individual client's needs. While there are inherent values and limitations of each assessment, these can be compounded or negated, depending on the psychosocial and health challenges of each patient. The following are some of the more common assessments, along with potential drawbacks and values of each one:

24-Hour Recall

Strengths are that it does not require literacy to complete, it is relatively simple and easy for the patient, it can be carried out via phone or in person, and data can be entered directly into the dietary analysis program. It is also useful for gathering information about meal patterning, food group intake, and can be used as a counseling tool. Limitations include the fact that it is based on self-reported information and is thus dependent on the patient's memory and honesty, it can be time consuming for the professional to analyze and also requires skill, and single recalls may not be representative of usual intake.

Food Frequency

Strengths are that it is inexpensive and easy to administer and complete, it can assess current and past diet, and, as a screening tool, it can provide a quick general overview for major dietary issues. Limitations include the fact that it cannot assess meal patterning and its use in the clinical setting is limited because it does not yield data about absolute intake for individuals.

Food Record

Strengths are that it can provide a fairly valid measure of meal patterning and nutrient intake, it does not require memory or recall, portions can be measured prior to consumption, and it can be used as a counseling tool. Limitations include the fact that it relies on self-reported data, it can be time consuming and burdensome to the patient and the nutrition staff, patients must be motivated and literate, staff need to be highly skilled at nutrition analysis, and the act of recording consumed foods can influence what is eaten.

Diet History

Strengths are that it does not require literacy to complete, it is appropriate for most patients, it can assess typical intake in a single interview session. It is also useful for gathering information about meal patterning, food group intake, and can be used as a counseling tool. Limitations are that the interview and post-interview analysis are quite time consuming, it relies on memory and honesty, and it requires a skilled interviewer to obtain complete, truthful data.

Methodology

Clinical data within a nutrition assessment provides medical history and current medical information which can include chronic or acute disease, use of prescription or over-the-counter medications, therapies, surgeries, as well as life stresses and daily routine. All of these factors can alter the absorption of key nutrients within the body, possibly leading to malnutrition and nutrient deficiencies, so it is important to make note of a patient's past and clinical information within the assessment. Evaluation of clinical data when reviewing an individual's nutrition assessment can help to uncover underlying causes of nutritional concerns. Of course, a professional must assess clinical data in addition to all other information within the assessment, including anthropometrics, diet history, psychosocial factors, and biochemical tests.

Documentation

Medical Charts

Accuracy is crucial when maintaining a medical chart. This chart is utilized by many different medical personnel on a daily basis, so it is very important that the chart be kept neat and organized. Documents must be placed in the correct section so that they can be easily located by medical personnel. Nutritional data will most likely be placed in the dietary section or progress notes section within the medical chart. In addition to the medical chart, the Minimum Data Set should be referenced. All information should be written legibly in blue or black ink. To correct a mistake, draw a single line through the text. Avoid scribbling or covering up previously recorded text. In some facilities, it may also be necessary to initial any changes made within the report.

Assessment Forms

The Minimum Data Set (MDS) is the federally mandated, standardized form used for a nutritional assessment. The MDS is included in the patient's medical chart and assesses the individual's physical, social, psychological, and emotional status. Section AC of the MDS form provides an overview of the patient's medical history followed by a list of questions pertaining to the individual's eating patterns and behaviors. Section K of the MDS form provides a more detailed explanation of the patient's oral and nutritional status. This section contains information on the subject of dietary intake, weight fluctuations, taste capabilities, and use of tube feeding devices of intravenous feeding.

Nutrition Assessment of Individuals

The first step in the Nutrition Care Process is to conduct a nutrition assessment on the individual. This assessment will evaluate the patient's nutritional requirements based on dietary intake, physical traits, biochemical data, medical history, and psychosocial factors. Dietary habits can be evaluated by conducting a diet history in order to identify insufficiencies, excesses, and changes. Anthropometric measurements include height, weight, Body Mass Index, and body fat percentages and are used to assess physical traits. Biochemical data consists of serum protein, vitamin, and mineral levels. These tests are based on blood or urine samples but can be distorted by certain medications, hydration status, or disease. Medical history is the clinical data of the individual encompassing acute or chronic disease, prescription or over-the-counter medications, or vitamin intake that may alter the nutritional needs of the patient. Evaluating psychosocial factors such as depression, anxiety, and other social issues will aid in determining whether these factors influence the individual's nutrient needs. The nutrition assessment is an important tool in the Nutrition Care Process of the individual and it is vital that all parts of the assessment be considered when preparing a plan of action for the nutritional care of the patient.

Anthropometric Data
An initial client assessment obtains current anthropometric data, such as height, weight, BMI, and circumference measurements. Caloric needs and metabolic rate are determined by body size and composition. Risk factors for various diseases such as cardiovascular disease and diabetes are affected by body fat and weight, so measuring these parameters is important. With children, growth charts are used to track relative height and weight and compare these values to standardized ones, to assess a child's percentile. For the greatest accuracy when tracking changes in weight, a client should be regularly weighed on the same calibrated physician's scale in similar conditions (time of day, clothing, eating status, etc.). Some examples of other common anthropometric assessments that nutrition professionals may conduct include the following:

Triceps Skin Fold Test
The triceps skin fold test is an anthropometric measurement technique that is performed in order to determine a patient's body fat percentage. Using a device called a caliper, the skin and fatty tissue are pinched and measured, avoiding the underlying muscle tissue. The site of the skinfold is found by determining the midpoint between the acromial process (top of the shoulder) and the olecranon process (back of the elbow) on the backside of the upper arm.

Waist to Hip Ratio
This determines the distribution of abdominal fat deposits. Evaluating measurements on this part of the body is very useful in predicting the risk of developing illnesses including cardiovascular disease and diabetes. To perform this assessment, a tape measure is used to measure the patient's waist at the narrowest part of the torso, usually directly above the navel. Next, the patient is measured around the widest part of the hips. Waist circumference is divided by hip circumference to determine the waist to hip ratio. In men, a WHR above 1.0 is considered at risk. For women, 0.8 or greater puts the patient at risk for developing certain diseases.

Arm Muscle Measurements
Arm muscle measurements are used in children in order to determine whether a child has sufficient skeletal muscle mass. This test can be useful in assessing nutritional status, particularly carbohydrates

and protein. If the child has a diet that is too low in carbohydrates, the body must accommodate by using protein for energy that would otherwise be used to build muscle mass.

Body Mass Index (BMI) $lb. \div inches^2 \times 703 = BMI$

Body mass index or BMI is a formula that uses height and weight in order to determine whether an individual is at a healthy weight. This formula is (kg)/[height (m)]2. A high BMI number can indicate a high percentage of adipose, or fatty, tissue in the body. A BMI chart is divided into sections in which a patient can fall: severely underweight (<17.4), underweight (17.5-18.4), normal weight (18.5-25), overweight (25.1-30), obese (30.1-40), and severely obese (>40.1). However, this number may be misleading as it does not account for muscle, skeletal, and water weight that makes up an individual's overall body composition.

Biochemical/Laboratory

Initial laboratory tests used for diagnosis of malnutrition and nutrition-related issues include a variety of hematological studies, urine analysis, and, depending on the patient, stool samples. It is important to get a general assessment of overall blood profile, protein status, electrolyte balance, and any nutritional deficiencies. Issues in any of these values may be indicative of inadequate or excessive intake or digestion and absorption issues.

Lab Abbreviations

Nutrition professionals should be familiar with the lab abbreviations for common biochemical assessments. Some of the more commonly encountered abbreviations for nutrition-related tests include the following:

- ALT; alanine transaminase, part of the liver function test (LFT)
- AST: alanine aminotransferase, part of the LFT
- BMP: basic metabolic panel
- BUN: blood urea nitrogen
- CBC: complete blood count, comprised of 15 different parameters
- CBL: cobalamin, vitamin B12
- CK: creatine phosphokinase (indicative of muscle damage)
- CMP: comprehensive metabolic panel
- HDL: high-density lipoprotein (cholesterol)
- LDL: low-density lipoprotein (cholesterol)
- CPR: C-Reactive Protein (elevated levels are indicative of inflammation)
- ESR: erythrocyte sedimentation rate
- INR: international normalized ratio (assesses if blood is clotting normally)
- LFT: liver function test
- WBC: white blood cell count
- RBC: red blood cell count
- HBC: hemoglobin
- HCT: hematocrit (percentage of red blood cells in circulation)
- PLT: platelets
- Trig: triglycerides
- TSH: thyroid stimulating hormone

Nutrition professionals should also be familiar with the measurement abbreviations that will appear on lab results. The following are several of the more common abbreviations:

- cmm: cells per cubic millimeter
- g/dL: grams per decliter
- IU: international units (often used as IU/L)
- Mg/dL: milligrams per deciliter
- pg: one-trillionth of a gram

Lab Values Related to and Indicative of Nutritional Status

Nutrition professionals should be familiar with the normal and abnormal ranges of the specific biochemical laboratory markers that are indicative of nutritional status. Most lab test results flag the client's values that fall outside of the normal ranges and report the actual value as well as the expected health range for each test, where available. While it is not necessary to memorize these ranges for this reason, it is helpful if nutrition professionals are comfortable reading lab results and have a familiarity with the specific tests to monitor for assessing nutritional status. The following chart lists some of the common tests and their reference ranges:

Biochemistry	Range	Haematology	Range
Albumin (g/l)	$27 - 39$	Haematocrit (%)	$24 - 46$
ALP (U/l)	$90 - 170$	Haemoglobin (g/dl)	$8 - 15$
BHB (mmol/l)	$0 - 1.2$	Lymphocytes ($10^9/l$)	$2.5 - 7.5$
CK (U/l)	$0 - 200$	Mean Cell HB (pg)	$11 - 17$
Cortisol* (ng/ml)	-	Mean Cell HB CN (g/dl)	$30 - 36$
Creatinine (µmol/l)	$44 - 165$	Mean Cell Volume (fl)	$40 - 60$
Fe (µmol/l)	$21 - 41$	Monocytes ($10^9/l$)	$0 - 0.8$
Fibronogen (g/l)	$2 - 5$	Neutrophils ($10^9/l$)	$0.6 - 4.0$
GGT (U/l)	$0 - 30$	Platelets ($10^9/l$)	$100 - 800$
Glucose (mmol/l)	$2.8 - 3.6$	RBC ($10^{12}/l$)	$5 - 10$
Haptoglobin (g/l)	$0 - 0.4$	White Cells ($10^9/l$)	$4 - 12$
NEFA (µmol/l)	$0 - 600$		
Total Protein (g/l)	$61 - 81$	Bands ($10^9/l$)	$0 - 0.1$
Transferrin* (%)	-	Basophils ($10^9/l$)	$0 - 0.2$
Triglycerides (mmol/l)	$0 - 20$	Eosinophils ($10^9/l$)	$0 - 2.0$
Urea (mmol/l)	$3.4 - 7.3$		
ZST (OD unit)	>20		

<u>Clinical</u>

Physical Assessments

There are a variety of physical assessments that can add value to nutrition consultations along with client history, medical history, BMI, and clinical data. The NFPT (Nutrition-Focused Physical Exam) is a full-body physical exam that nutrition professionals can use to assess nutritional status, signs of malnutrition, deficiency, or nutrient toxicity. Body symmetry, breathing, posture, frailty, emotional status, communication ability, shape, texture, color of fingernails, skin color and texture, hair, eyes, odors, and body shape should all be assessed. Blood pressure is an easy, non-invasive biomarker that can shed light on overall trends in health for the individual. For example, with hypertensive clients referred to nutrition management for health improvements, monitoring blood pressure improvements over baseline with a dietary intervention can help clients gain self-efficacy and motivation that the work they are putting in is improving their health. Diets such as the DASH diet are specifically designed to improve heart health and blood pressure, so monitoring blood pressure is particularly important with this plan. For all clients, it is important to take a general physical inventory of signs and symptoms of nutritional influences on health and wellbeing. Digestive symptoms can be indicative of food intolerances or allergies, as can rashes, headaches, fatigue after eating, and joint pain. Other physical signs such as brittle nails, temperature intolerance, difficulty sleeping, moodiness, lethargy, and a weakened immune system can be signs of nutritional deficiencies and may indicate the need for further laboratory analysis.

Medical History

A full medical history can provide nutrition professionals with a detailed picture of overall health, which is necessary to begin developing a suitable plan and nutrition goals. Medical history useful to nutrition professionals includes immunizations, surgeries, hospitalizations, major illnesses or injuries, current or recent prescriptions, vitamin/mineral/herbal supplements, over-the-counter medications, laxatives, any known allergies and food allergies. Certain medications can have interactions with nutrients, such as potassium-wasting diuretics. Family history and current health statuses of immediate family members is also important because certain diseases such as diabetes, heart disease, hypertension, and hypercholesteremia can have a genetic component.

Physical Activity

Independent of a healthy diet, physical activity reduces the risk of several chronic diseases and improves overall health. According to the U.S. General's recommendations, children should participate in sixty minutes of moderate to vigorous physical activity daily, and adults should accumulate a minimum of thirty minutes of moderate to vigorous activity on most, if not all, days per week. Nutrition professionals should gather information about exercise patterns, type, intensity, duration, and preferences. In addition to focusing on exercise, it is important to also discuss general daily life activity patterns such as energy demands of the occupation, commuting method and duration, time spent sedentary, and responsibilities regarding home care or childcare. Not only do activity patterns and intensity affect caloric needs, but they also impact food timing, disease risk factors, and overall health profile. For those patients who are physically inactive, proper education on the importance of daily exercise should be provided and a referral to an allied health professional in the fitness industry may be prudent.

Medications/Nutrient Interactions

Certain commonly used medications can lead to adverse side effects. For example, aspirin may cause gastrointestinal bleeding, leading to the loss of iron in the body. This medication can also interfere with the balance and uptake of ascorbic acid, or Vitamin C, causing increased excretion in the urine, and therefore decreased amounts available for use in the body. In extreme cases, aspirin may lead to gastric ulcerations.

Diuretics are often prescribed to treat symptoms of a variety of conditions including diabetes, kidney disease or kidney stones, polycystic ovary disease, edema, heart failure, and osteoporosis. However, they carry a risk of certain potentially serious side effects. Depending on the type of diuretic, too much or too little potassium in the blood may result. Diuretics can increase the absorption of calcium in the intestine, leading to excretion of potassium, sodium, and magnesium through the urine.

Corticosteroids, such as prednisone and hydrocortisone, are beneficial in the treatment of asthma, lupus, allergies, and rashes. They can be administered orally, topically, by way of an inhaler, or via an injection. Side effects include decreased calcium absorption, decreased protein synthesis, eye problems such as glaucoma or cataracts, high blood pressure, fluid retention, weight gain, and psychological effects as well as decreased bone formation, increased excretion of potassium and nitrogen, and an increased need for Vitamin D.

Other examples of commonly prescribed medications that carry adverse side effects include antidepressants and MAOI drugs. Use of antidepressants can disrupt sodium distribution in the body. MAOI drugs can lead to an increase in appetite with subsequent weight gain.

Medical Terminology monoamine oxidase inhibitors (m AOI)

Registered dietetic technicians should familiarize themselves with basic medical terminology, as this will improve their ability to effectively communicate with referring physicians and other allied health professionals. It is expected that registered dietetic technicians will communicate regularly with the medical professionals overseeing, coordinating, and delivering healthcare to their shared clients. Using the appropriate medical terminology improves the credibility of the nutrition professional and understanding such language will certainly facilitate a greater understanding during conversations, which will ultimately lead to better patient care.

Nutrition Intake

Although seemingly obvious, obtaining accurate and thorough data regarding a client's nutrition intake is essential to accurate dietary analysis and meal plan formulation. While the specific nutrient focus may vary for each individual client, such as attention to iron intake for an anemic client or simple sugar consumption for a patient with diabetes, complete and honest records should be obtained from every client. It is important to have a thorough picture of nutrition intake for proper assessment and planning for every patient. Depending on the goals and needs of the patient, nutrition intake may need reassessment at regular intervals or with changing health conditions or concerns.

Assessment Method

Having a healthy diet can improve clients' energy, weight management, exercise performance, sleep quality, and mental focus—all of which contribute to a higher fitness level as well as improved overall health and quality of life. Throughout the training process, trainers should regularly review their clients' diets and emphasize getting consistent, quality nutrition. Clients can report their dietary habits in any of the following ways:

24-Hour Recall

Twenty-four hour recalls are recordings of all consumed meals, snacks, and beverages in a twenty-four-hour period, their quantities, and preparation methods. It is easy to obtain and most clients can readily report the consumption in the previous day in a first encounter appointment, without having prepared logs or journals. However, it is limited in its overall representation of an average or long-term dietary habits of the patient, and estimating quantities can be difficult for patients, especially for restaurant foods.

Food Frequency Questionnaire

Food frequency questionnaires are detailed reports that delve into dietary habits and identify possible triggers associated with less healthy habits based on questionnaires about how often and in what quantities certain food groups and beverages are consumed in daily, weekly, and monthly patterns. Benefits of this method are that it evaluates long-term dietary habits and can identify inadequate intake of any food groups, and thus, possible deficiencies. Disadvantages are that it does not examine food preparation methods, and patients may not include or lower the frequencies reported of unhealthy foods.

Diet History

Diet history is made up of recordings of all consumed meals, snacks, and beverages in a twenty-four-hour period, three-day, or seven-day log. Benefits of this method are that it evaluates long-term dietary habits and is quick and easy. Disadvantages are that it can be hard for a patient to record a "typical" daily intake if diet is varied, and patients may not include or lower the frequencies reported of unhealthy foods.

In order to evaluate the nutritional habits and routines of the patient, it is important to utilize a diet history. Doing so will help to locate certain nutritional deficiencies or excesses within the diet. The diet history is a series of interview questions concerning food intake over the last few (usually three to seven) days. The interviewer may initially start by obtaining a 24-hour recall of food intake from the patient. Next, a food frequency questionnaire is completed followed by a food journal, documenting intake over several weekdays and a weekend day. The diet history should cover food preparation methods in addition to what types of foods were consumed. There should also be information pertaining to any disabilities, allergies, or recent medical therapies that may hinder a patient's ability to prepare or consume certain foods. The patient may have cultural or religious beliefs that prevent them from eating some foods, and this should be noted in the diet history as well. Use of prescription or over-the-counter pharmaceuticals and supplements must also be recorded considering that these could alter the patient's nutritional status by interfering with or altering the absorption of vitamins and minerals.

Fluid Status (I/Os)

Hydration status of clients can be assessed by comparing input and output and determining fluid status and possible dehydration. Elderly clients and those with chronic illnesses are especially likely to suffer from dehydration. Aging leads to decreased lean body mass and, over time, decreased body water. Seniors may also be at risk for dehydration because of decreased sensitivity to thirst and diminished ability of the kidneys to concentrate urine in the absence of adequate hydration. Dehydration is a loss of at least 1% of body mass due to fluid loss. Dehydration can affect metabolic processes, cognitive function, mood, energy, and organ function. Fluid intake comes from dietary fluid and food intake and output is from urine, sweat, respiration, and fecal matter.

Interviews/Verification

The interviewer must take great care to conduct the diet history interview with the patient in such a way that they are not intimidating or leading the patient to answer a question in a particular way. Before the interview, matters such as language barriers, hearing loss, or other communication issues that could present a challenge should be planned for. A translator, family member, or caretaker should attend the interview so that any communication problems can be taken care of. It may also be a good idea for the patient to have someone else present during the interview if that patient suffers from memory loss or dementia.

It is important to phase questions appropriately when performing a diet history interview. Positive language should be used at all times and accusatory tones should be avoided. Questions should be asked in such a way that the interviewer comes across as simply looking to gather information, as opposed to criticizing the patient's eating habits. The interviewer should ask: "How many sugar sweetened drinks do you consume each day?" rather than, "You don't drink sugary beverages every day, do you?" It is also important for the interviewer to consider the responses to the patient's answers very carefully. For example, if a patient states that he or she does, in fact, consume an abundance of sugary beverages throughout the day, the interview is not the time or place to offer opinions or counseling to the patient on any particular issue. The interviewer is simply gathering information to be evaluated and developed into a plan of action at a later time.

Analysis of Dietary Information

After all nutrient intake data is collected during the assessment process, the actual analysis of the dietary information begins. This process requires careful, meticulous work and significant skill on behalf of the nutrition professional. Thankfully, with the development and refinement of various dietary analysis software programs in recent years, this process has become more efficient and automated, reducing both the physical and mental energy required from staff. Even with sophisticated software or online databases, nutrition professionals have to know how to calculate the dietary information from foods that do not contain a nutrition label, such as those from home-cooked meals, recipes, restaurant offerings, and caloric beverages, such as smoothies and blended coffee drinks. Cooking preparations, portion sizes, and the conversion from a purchased portion to the edible portion from any recipe or meal must all be considered. In addition to the thorough analysis of macronutrient intake and ratios (including amino acid profile, fiber intake, and type and proportions of various fatty acids and lipids), micronutrients—including vitamins and minerals—must be assessed. Deficiencies and excesses can lead to impaired immunity, metabolism, growth, and health. In some cases, the timing of food intake should be considered during the analysis process. For example, meal timing affects blood glucose levels, which is especially important for patients with diabetes. The absorption of certain micronutrients is augmented or hindered by the consumption of other concurrent nutrients. For example, iron absorption is enhanced with the intake of vitamin C but restricted when ingested with calcium-containing foods.

Oral Dietary Supplements

Oral dietary supplements, including vitamins, minerals, herbs, and even some medicines, should be included in the analysis of dietary intake. Patients may be taking isolated or multivitamin and mineral supplements, omega 3 fatty acids, probiotics, calcium, iron, magnesium, or folate, vitamin C, B-12 or a general B complex, among many others. Some supplements—particularly herbal tinctures—are not regulated by the FDA, and therefore do not contain detailed product labels, and may even lack ingredient lists. In some cases, contacting the manufacturer can yield useful product information, but other times, an approximate estimation is the best that can be done. While supplementation may be necessary for clients with certain medical conditions or who follow restricted diets, it is recommended that nutrient intake comes from food sources whenever possible. The bioavailability of nutrients in oral supplements is somewhat unknown, although most research indicates that it is inferior to whole food sources. Certain formulations and sources may be superior to others; studies from independent companies typically yield the most unbiased data.

Enteral Feeding

Enteral feeding is an option for patients who cannot tolerate oral feedings, usually due to an inability to chew or decreased peristalsis. With this type of feeding, food is delivered directly into the stomach using a feeding tube. The type of feeding tube and placement of the tube, either on the stomach or somewhere along the gastro-intestinal tract, can vary from patient to patient. Proper sanitation techniques are very important when caring for a patient undergoing enteral tube feeding because there is a direct line from the outside environment to the stomach, putting the patient at a much greater risk of infection.

Enteral Feeding Formulas TF/EN uses digestive system via GI or stomach

In order for enteral tube feeding to be successful, the patient must have two or more feet of properly functioning small intestine. Enteral feeding formulas may be commercially or individually prepared. Commercially prepared formulas are more convenient, consistent in nutrient content, and cost less, while individually prepared formulas are tailored to the needs of each patient. Formulae are prepared using water, carbohydrates, fat, protein, vitamins, and minerals in varying amounts. To reduce costs and increase trace nutrient content, formulae can also be prepared using whole foods that have been pureed and strained; however, this method increases the risk of contamination and requires a larger feeding tube. Most enteral formulas provide 1 – 1.5 kcals/cc, and glucose provides carbohydrates, amino acids provide protein, and monoglycerides provide lipids.

Possible Complications

There are several problems that may occur in patients undergoing enteral feeding. Frequent diarrhea (more than three bowel movements per day), is a sign that there is a problem with the feeding system or the patient is not tolerating the enteral tube feeding. Patients should be screened for lactose intolerance and given lactose-free formula, if necessary. Additionally, enteral formulae must be discarded and switched out every day in order to decrease the risk of bacterial contamination. A continuous drip method can help if the formula has a high osmolality or if the formula is being infused too rapidly. Nausea and vomiting can be a sign that the gastrointestinal tract is not functioning properly, in which case the feeding tube should be repositioned into the duodenum. If this does not stop the nausea and vomiting, parental feeding may be necessary. Elevating the patient's head during feeding or switching to a smaller tube or repositioning the tube into the duodenum can help to prevent aspiration, which puts the patient at risk of pneumonia. Frequent flushing of the feeding tube or switching to a larger tube can help to prevent obstruction of the tube.

Parenteral Feeding   TF into bloodstream - bypass digestive system

TPN
PPN

Parenteral feeding is used if the gut is no longer functioning because this feeding method delivers nutrients directly into the bloodstream via a catheter, completely bypassing the digestive system. The increased risk of infection is a concern for patients receiving parenteral nutrition, so proper sanitation techniques must be followed. Similar to enteral feedings, the formulas that are delivered to the patient will vary in nutrient composition, depending on the individual need of the patient.

Parenteral Formulas amino acids, lipids + dextrose

In order for protein synthesis and anabolism to occur, the parenteral solution should provide 1 gram of protein per 150 calories, unless the patient in severely weakened, in which case the solution should be adjusted to 1 gram per 100 calories. Protein is provided from amino acids and most solutions will range from 5 to 15 percent amino acids, but can be adjusted depending on the disease state. Carbohydrates are provided in the form of dextrose and should be administered at a rate of no more than 4 to 5 mg/kg/minute, in order to prevent hyperglycemia and excessive carbon dioxide production and 25 to 35 percent of calories should come from lipids to prevent fatty acid deficiency. Potassium and phosphorus levels will also need to be monitored.

Transitional Feeding

Transitional feeding refers to the period of time when a patient moves from one method of feeding to another. This could be moving from parenteral to enteral to oral or enteral to oral feeding methods.

Transitioning between feeding methods must be done slowly and monitored closely because patients who have gone without solid foods for a long period of time are at risk of hypophosphatemia, as phosphorus can move out of the plasma and enter the cells at a very rapid pace if the transition back to oral feeding is too aggressive. Alcoholics, diabetics, and kidney disease patients are at a greater risk of developing this complication, and phosphate supplementation may be necessary. It is also important to monitor potassium levels in patients going through feeding method transitions. The first meals should be lactose-free, due to the fact that enzyme counts are low following a period of enteral or parenteral feeding methods, so the patient may not be able to digest lactose. This can then be reintroduced gradually. The first meals should also be low in sodium and carbohydrates and supplemented with electrolytes.

Economic/Social

Socioeconomic
Migrants and Homeless Individuals
Migrant families and homeless individuals lead lives that make it very difficult for nutritional care. The frequent location changes of migrants means that medical records must travel with them, which may result in missing vital information. It is important that medical professionals communicate across different communities in order to keep medical documents up to date and organized for migrant families. Nutritional counseling and education can also be a challenge due to language barriers and cultural differences.

Homeless individuals suffer from a number of barriers that make proper nutrition a challenge. Financial issues hinder their ability to purchase healthy foods, and many social service programs are not able to provide them with nutritionally balanced meals. They may not be able to accommodate infants and children at all. Programs like WIC offer support for these families, but lack of transportation presents another challenge. In most cases, homeless individuals cannot store or prepare foods properly and safely. With larger families on tight budgets, the financial viability of healthy food choices may be limited, and the affordability of unhealthy alternatives often presents a more attractive alternative. An increasing number of green markets and Community Supported Agriculture (CSA) shares accept food stamps or offer subsidized produce. Nutrition professionals should research the available healthy options in their local areas so they can properly educate clients.

Cultural/Religious Food Patterns
Certain cultural and religious food practices may affect dietary intake and nutrition planning for certain clients. For example, kosher practices govern the intake of certain food groups within one meal, and all food must be blessed or certified Kosher. Various religious groups avoid certain meats, and celebratory and special food practices can affect food preferences and dietary intake. Those who are Seventh Day Adventists likely do not consume any animal products and may need vitamin B-12 supplementation. Nutrition professionals should be sensitive to different cultural and religious food patterns, while still striving to help improve the dietary health of their clients.

Native American and Alaskan Native Populations
The Native American and Alaskan native population has seen a dramatic increase in obesity rates in recent years and, in turn, an increase in obesity-related diseases such as heart disease, diabetes, and hypertension. A number of factors have contributed to the rise in health risk of this population. Individuals have moved away from traditional foods like venison, buffalo, leaner meats, plant-based foods, and complex carbohydrates in favor of a high fat, high sugar, and fast food diet. On reservations,

there is easy access to sugary drinks, processed meats, and refined carbohydrates. In addition to obesity-related diseases, tooth decay and alcoholism are also prevalent.

Psychological/Behavioral

Certain psychological and behavioral practices can affect dietary intake. Depression, anxiety, sleep disturbances, and even hectic work schedules can negatively affect food choices, caloric intake, and appetite. When it seems that such issues are impacting diet or other healthy behaviors, nutrition professionals should refer clients to mental health professionals for support. Eating disorders are also complex psychological disorders that significantly affect nutrient intake.

Disordered eating behaviors include binge eating, abnormal or obsessive dieting, regularly skipping meals, self-induced vomiting, calorie counting to a level that is obsessive, having a self-worth tied to physique, misusing diuretics and laxatives, and unhealthy fasting or restrictive eating. The root cause of an eating disorder may vary from one individual to another, but it is believed that eating disorders can be attributed to genetics, environmental, social, and cultural factors. An eating disorder is a mental illness with a set of specific diagnostic criteria as described in the *Diagnostic and Statistical Manual of Mental Disorders* (DSM) published by the American Psychiatric Association, a professional association of psychiatric physicians. The most recent version of the DSM is the DSM-5, published in 2013, and it specifies four types of eating disorders: anorexia nervosa (AN), bulimia nervosa (BN), binge eating disorder (BED), and other eating disorders.

Anorexia Nervosa Subtypes: (1) restricting (2.) binge eating

Anorexia nervosa (AN) is characterized by consistently restricting caloric intake to keep body weight at least 15 percent lower than would be healthy for age, sex, development, and health; an intense fear of becoming overweight or obese; and having a distorted self-image of body weight or shape. Historically, AN has been more prevalent in females, although more recent studies indicate that adolescent females and males suffer from the disease equally. AN can further be classified into two subtypes: restricting and binge eating. Individuals who exhibit behavior of restricting AN limit certain food groups and/or their amounts, obsessively count calories, skip meals, and are obsessive in their attempt to adhere to guidance and rules governing consumption. Individuals with AN who exhibit binge eating behavior may also restrict certain food groups and quantities, but also display binging and purging behaviors. Binge eating involves eating a large amount of food and feeling a sense of loss of control while doing so; purging involves self-induced tactics to rid the body of food such as vomiting; using laxatives, diuretics, and enemas; or participating in excessive exercise.

Bulimia Nervosa Subtypes (1) purging (2.) non-purging

In bulimia nervosa (BN), similar to AN, individuals typically have a distorted self-image of body shape, weight, or size. Other behaviors characterized by BN include binge eating large amounts of food while feeling a sense of lack of control, self-induced vomiting, and misusing laxatives, diuretics, or enemas to prevent weight gain. In individuals with BN, the binge eating behavior occurs at least weekly for three months. Bulimia nervosa can further be categorized into purging and non-purging type behavior. Purging behaviors involve tactics to remove food from the body, while non-purging behaviors involve restricting food or engaging in excessive exercise to compensate for food that has been ingested.

Binge Eating Disorder

Binge eating disorder (BED) is characterized by persistent binge eating, feeling a sense of distress when binging, or binging on average weekly for three months. Binge eating is closely related to BN, but individuals do not engage in purging or other compensatory behaviors that would eliminate food from their bodies.

Other Eating Disorders

Other eating disorders are now classified in the DSM-5 as other specified feeding or eating disorder (OSFED) or unspecified feeding or eating disorder (UFED). These two categories are intended to recognize disordered eating behaviors that do not clearly align with other diagnosed and defined eating disorders. Night eating syndrome, which entails recurrent episodes of eating at night, is one example of an OSFED.

Effects of Eating Disorders on the Body

Physiological changes can occur as a result of disordered eating, putting individuals at risk for other health issues. Physical signs and symptoms that may be associated with AN and its behaviors include rapid weight loss, mineral and electrolyte imbalances, amenorrhea in females, decreased sex drive, fainting or dizziness, hypothermia, consistently feeling cold even in warm weather, bloating, constipation, food intolerances, fatigue, low energy level, changes in the face including sunken eyes, and the development of fine hair on the face and body. Health concerns associated with AN and its behaviors include anemia, immune compromise, gastrointestinal issues, amenorrhea in females, increased risk of infertility in men and women, renal failure, osteoporosis, cardiovascular issues, and ultimately, death.

Signs and symptoms that may be associated with BN include frequent change in weight; physical signs associated with vomiting including facial swelling, knuckle calluses, tooth decay, and bad breath; chronic sore throat; bloating, constipation, and food intolerances; amenorrhea; fainting or dizziness; and tiredness. Health concerns associated with BN include dehydration; gastrointestinal reflux, heartburn, and ulcers; slowed or irregular heartbeat; electrolyte imbalances; and heart failure.

BED can lead to weight gain and obesity, high blood pressure, high cholesterol, kidney failure, osteoarthritis, diabetes, stroke, gallbladder disease, irregular menstrual cycle, skin disorders, heart disease, and some cancers.

As a result of disordered eating, individuals can develop physiological issues that lead to health problems. These health problems can lead to a variety of conditions that can compromise health and even lead to death. Children and adolescents who develop disordered eating are at even greater risk of injury and physiological complications, since growth and development may be affected by disordered eating. Females, particularly athletes, are also at risk for the Female Athlete Triad—a combination of energy deficiency and/or disordered eating, irregular menstrual cycles or amenorrhea, and osteoporosis or bone mineral loss.

Lifestyles/Preferences

Lifestyle and preferences significantly impact food choices. Lifestyle factors to consider include, but are not limited to, access to healthy food, work schedule, comfort with and time dedicated to cooking, kitchen equipment, childcare or elder care responsibilities, physical activity interest, and leisure activity preferences.

Food Fads/Cultism

With diet and weight-loss related products comprising a multi-billion-dollar industry annually, it is imperative that the effective registered dietetic technician is familiar with the most popular and prevalent "fad" diets that clients could possibly attempt. Many clients are intrigued by the promise of "quick fixes" that many popularized diets purport, and may enter nutrition counseling with a greater interest in attempting one of these such methods over the more sound scientifically based nutritional guidance that the registered dietetic professional has to offer. Nutrition professionals should prepare easily understood pamphlets or other resources that can explain the dangers of "fad" diets and the fallacies in many of the stated claims. Understanding the benefits of and principles behind the recommended nutritional program and the issues with fad diets may make it easier for clients to adhere to the healthy nutritional and lifestyle changes advised by their registered dietetic technician.

Level of Education

A client's level of education can have a significant impact on the counseling process as well as the delivery and effectiveness of a nutritional program. With math skills and language comprehension, nutrition professionals should be able to deliver nutrition program components in a way that is understandable to the client, so that the client can comprehend and implement the program successfully. Clients whose level of education poses limitations on understanding or applying information may require more guidance or additional resources. Registered dietetic technicians should consider the client's ability to comprehend guidelines, restrictions, and recommendations when choosing the most appropriate and useful tools, resources, and easy-to-understand information. Doing so will increase the likelihood of the client's commitment and adherence to the suggested program.

Nutrition Knowledge and Interest

Clients who have more nutrition knowledge and a background in paying attention to diet, reading food labels, and prioritizing healthy eating are often quite motivated to take on recommended programs and can usually jump into programs at an advanced level, with less instruction. Even clients who lack experience or education paying attention to diet can be engaged and motivated, particularly if they are excited about improving their health. With a vested interest in the nutrition programming process, a client also has a higher probability of achieving success in his or her health goals. While a client's knowledge of and interest in nutrition can be helpful for nutrition professionals working with them, even clients who lack knowledge and interest can be easily informed with resources such as websites, visual aids, etc. that explain the necessity of proper nutrition for health and provide tips on how to seamlessly integrate a nutrition program into daily life.

Needs Assessment

Nutrition professionals should conduct a needs assessment prior to working with a new individual client and also when planning programming for a population. Time constraints, financial limitations, medical restrictions, and family responsibilities are examples of external constraints that can affect, or even sabotage, a client's adherence to a recommended nutrition program. For example, financial limitations should be considered when recommending food choices for a family with a very limited income. Internal constraints, like illness or lack of knowledge or motivation, can also affect program adherence and necessary program components. With pertinent information relating to the client's concerns and constraints, the program can be structured to optimize success. For example, limitations with respect to time, food availability, or mobility can all be addressed and resolved with proper planning.

When designing programs for populations, needs assessments are crucial; they not only help identify necessary program components, but they also uncover barriers that must be addressed in the planning stages in order to implement a successful program. USDA's federal assistance WIC programs are implemented in new communities after conducting large-scale needs assessments on each new community. For example, extensive surveys are distributed to identify literacy levels so educational materials are appropriate. Similarly, the need for breastfeeding education is assessed by estimating the percentage of new or expectant mothers planning to breastfeed.

<u>Educational Readiness Assessment</u>

When preparing a client to engage in the necessary steps required to produce an effective nutrition program, the nutrition professional should first perform an educational readiness assessment to determine how best to approach the topics of nutrition and the steps involved in applying the nutrition program to daily life. In evaluating a client's levels of education and motivation, the nutrition professional should also evaluate the environmental and social factors that may impact the successful implementation of the nutrition program.

Motivational Level

A client's motivational level is essential in his or her desire to adhere to the prescribed program. The motivation behind the reason for which the client is seeking nutrition services is also important to assess. Some clients may approach nutrition professionals to improve health or disease risk factors, others may be medically referred for disease conditions or failure to grow properly, some desire aesthetic improvements or athletic gains, while others are looking to lose weight or increase fertility. While all clients may be motivated to follow the advice and programming provided, those who are highly motivated tend to be more successful in implementing the health and nutrition program elements provided.

When individuals need to change their behavior, it's important to understand that change is a process and that individuals often move through six stages referred to as the *trans theoretical model of behavior change*: precontemplation, contemplation, preparation, action, maintenance, and termination. During the precontemplation stage, individuals are not really thinking about making any changes, do not see their behavior as problematic, and are typically not ready for change. When individuals are in the contemplation stage, they recognize there is a problem, are thinking about making a change, and usually getting ready to make change. During the preparation stage, individuals are ready to make a change and may actually begin making small changes in their behavior. During the action phase, individuals are making consistent apparent changes in their behavior. In the maintenance stage, individuals have made changes for a sustained period, usually six months or longer, and are working to prevent any setbacks. During the final stage of change—termination—individuals have sustained the maintenance stage for quite some time and have no desire to return to their previous behaviors. Nutrition professionals need to be aware of these stages of change when working with individuals who need to change their diet and health behaviors.

Educational Level

The education level of a client can impact his or her adherence to a nutrition program and how well he or she is able to understand and apply the information provided about nutrition and health. Nutrition professionals should ask and also assess a client's understanding of basic nutrition science, macronutrients and micronutrients, caloric needs and caloric density of foods, portion sizes, the benefits of nutritious foods, and the impact of a healthy diet on overall health. A client who has or receives education from the nutrition professional is able to implement the advice and elements of a nutritional program more easily than those without. Clients who need education on the basics of nutrition, reading food labels, assessing nutritious elements of meals, etc. will require a more in-depth approach to their nutrition program, particularly at the beginning of the program. Identifying the client's general education level—including reading and math skills—can help the nutrition professional determine the most effective way to present information to the client to ensure understanding. For example, it may be inappropriate to give a client who does not have the equivalent of a high school education a complicated research journal article about omega 3 fatty acids or expect him or her to calculate macronutrient percentages of daily meals. Tailoring reference materials, verbal education, and the presentation of the program toward the educational level of a client will help prevent frustration and promote adherence.

Situational

Restrictions placed upon clients due to their environmental and economical situations can have a major impact on their adherence to a proposed program. Nutrition professionals should inquire about financial limitations (such as those that limit the client's ability to purchase or prepare healthy foods), time restrictions that may make preparing healthy meals an issue, or even environmental issues, such as family involvement, which can place healthy lifestyle and diet choices in the hands of people who may be less supportive of healthy and nutritious choices. Providing resources to clients in need can assist them in managing situational restrictions effectively.

Target Groups and Populations 1st identify target group then assess demographics

In order to design the most effective nutrition program, nutrition professionals should always consider the target group or population for which the program is being provided. Because different populations likely have varying needs and interests, identifying the group and then assessing their demographic and physical characteristics through questionnaires, interviews, and surveys can enable nutrition professionals to design effective programs for the group. For example, the needs and interests of women hoping to get pregnant are going to be different than those of school age children who are overweight and need to make dietary changes. Programs will be more clinically and financially successful if they are tailored to a specific group.

Nutrition Assessment of Populations

Nutritional assessments can serve as useful tools that provide insight into the needs of certain populations. By identifying the areas of need in a specific population, new approaches can be developed to provide the needed education, information, and programs designed specifically to reduce or eliminate the issues identified for the target population. Populations can be predetermined to include those belonging to a specific sex, age group, culture, or environment, which can help organize, identify, and provide the most effective resources. Because populations can be large, surveys and other large-scale assessment methods are often more cost- and time-efficient than conducting data on a one-by-one basis.

Nutrition Status Indicators

In the pediatric population, the most common nutrition status indicators are the CDC's weight and height charts. These are used to track the growth of children compared to reference data and ensure that the child is maintaining an adequate rate of growth over time and relative to that which is expected of his or her age. Body Mass Index (BMI) is also used for children and adults. Absolute or relative (percentile) BMI can classify an individual as underweight, normal weight, overweight, or obese. Stature-for-age from the growth charts is also used for this purpose. For example, those whose stature-for-age is lower than the 5th percentile are considered of short stature; similarly, a BMI falling in the lowest 5th percentile is categorized as underweight.

Age, Sex, Ethnic, and Cultural Groups

The Elderly

There many factors that people face as they age that can affect their ability to consume a healthy diet. As mentioned, sense of taste, smell, and sight may decrease, which can impair eating habits. Elderly patients normally consume a number of different medications, some of which can lead to food tasting metallic or losing flavor altogether. Mastication may become difficult for older adults as they are at increased risk of tooth decay or may have issues with ill-fitting dentures. In this case, soft or liquid foods may need to replace foods that are difficult to chew. Swallowing can also become difficult due to decreased salivary and esophageal function. The digestive tract commonly begins to lose function and motility, leading to digestive complications such as constipation or nauseas when eating.

In addition to these physical issues observed in elderly patients, concerns such as dementia or depression can lead to decreased nutritional status. Elderly individuals may have difficulties travelling to the grocery store or preparing healthy meals for themselves, especially those who live alone. Financial issues can also affect older adults as they stop working, leading to the inability to purchase healthy foods.

Specific Needs Populations

Pregnancy
Nutritional intervention is crucial for women before, during, and after pregnancy. Dietary needs change significantly during pregnancy, so it is important for women to monitor their diets for their own health as well as their baby's.

The need for Vitamin D doubles from 5 micrograms to 10 micrograms per day during pregnancy, due to the fact that it is so important for fetal skeletal formation. This vitamin is also crucial in the regulation of calcium metabolism, which increases during pregnancy. Vitamin D can be difficult to obtain through a regular diet. Food sources, such as milk, must be supplemented with Vitamin D, in order for the general public to reach the recommended amounts though food. Other sources include regular exposure to sunlight or supplementation.

Folic Acid, another essential nutrient for a healthy pregnancy, is a vitamin that is necessary for the production of new cells in the body and for synthesis of nucleic acids, which are the building blocks of DNA. It is important for women of childbearing age to start to building up adequate stores of folic acid even before becoming pregnant. This will greatly reduce the risk of certain birth defects, including brain or spine malformations. This vitamin can be obtained through the diet from food sources such as leafy green vegetables, fruits, enriched breads and cereals, nuts, and beans. In addition, folic acid supplement can be used to reach the recommended amounts of this vitamin. The RDA for women aged thirteen and up is 400 micrograms per day. This increases to 600 micrograms daily for pregnant women and 500 micrograms for breastfeeding women.

Iron recommendations during pregnancy doubles from 15 milligrams to 30 milligrams per day. This mineral is important in the function of red blood cells, the formation of which increases dramatically during pregnancy. Iron is essential for the growth of the fetus and development of the placenta. Food sources of iron include red meats, legumes, and spinach. Supplementation may also be necessary in order to reach the recommended amounts that will help to prevent premature delivery and low birth weight.

Children and Pregnant Women
To assure that low income pregnant women, infants, and children receive the assistance they need to stay healthy, the Centers for Disease Control and Prevention (CDC) has implemented two major programs to monitor this need. The Pediatric Nutrition Surveillance System (PedNSS) and The Pregnancy Nutrition Surveillance System (PNSS) have been put in place in order to monitor and assess the nutritional status of these populations. The Pediatric Nutrition Surveillance System compiles data from social service programs that provide health care, supplemental nutrition, and nutrition education to infants and children from low-income families. The Special Supplemental Nutrition Program for Women,

Infants, and Children (WIC), Early Periodic Screening, Diagnosis, and Treatment Programs (EPSDT), and Title V Maternal and Child Health Program (MCH) are among the federally funded health care programs from which this data is pulled. This information is then used to analyze current programs and implement new public health policies based on nutrition-related indicators including birth weight, stature, and body mass index.

The Pregnancy Nutrition Surveillance System (PNSS) focuses on the health of low-income pregnant women. A woman's nutritional status during her pregnancy will determine the overall health of the child, so it is important to gather information on topics such as maternal weight gain, prenatal vitamin intake, anemia, hypertension, smoking or drinking during pregnancy, and diabetes in order to develop health policies. Data is pulled from existing public health programs including the Special Supplemental Nutrition Program for Women, Infants, and Children (WIC) and Title V Maternal and Child Health Program (MCH). Information gathered from these programs can help to develop public health policies that will decrease the risk of premature deliveries, low birth weights, and birth defects.

Common Dietary Modifications
Just as in the general population, pregnant women should be encouraged to follow a well balanced diet that is rich in fruits, vegetables, whole grains, and lean meats. On average, calorie intake should increase between 220 and 400 more per day, depending on pre-pregnancy weight and overall health status of the woman. Pregnant women should monitor their intake of vitamins and mineral, particularly their increased need for vitamin D, calcium, folic acid, and iron. Although there are many food sources of these nutrients, a prenatal multivitamin should be used in most cases to ensure the patient is receiving adequate amounts. Hydration needs also increase with pregnancy due to fluid stores being used up more quickly, so consuming at least eight glasses of water per day is important. Pregnant women should also take care to avoid certain foods and beverages such as alcohol, liver, and seafood high in mercury, including shark, swordfish, mackerel, and tilefish.

Supplementing a Pregnant Woman's Diet
Even the healthiest, most well balanced diet during pregnancy may still fall short of providing sufficient amounts of recommended nutrients. A prenatal vitamin should be encouraged for pregnant women to ensure they obtain all the nutrients necessary to have a healthy pregnancy and delivery for herself and her baby.

Nutrition Risk Factors tx- eat ↑ Fe Foods or supplements
Iron Deficiency - anemia; lack of healthy red blood cells
Iron is an important mineral used in the body to transfer oxygen to the lungs. Iron deficiency is a common problem that can be easily reversed, in most cases, by increasing the amount of iron rich foods in the diet. If not treated, iron deficiency may lead to anemia, a condition in which the body is lacking in healthy red blood cells. Symptoms of low iron include fatigue, impaired immune function, inability to regulate body temperature, and slow development. Increasing consumption of Vitamin C in the diet will help as well, since this vitamin aids in the absorption of iron into the blood stream. Some food sources of iron include red meat, nuts, seafood, beans, leafy greens, and liver. Iron deficiency can develop due to rapid growth, large amounts of blood loss, and pregnancy.

Celiac Disease tx- avoid Gluten / B-vitamin supplements
Celiac disease is an autoimmune disorder in which the individual is reactive to gluten, a type of structural protein found in wheat and grains such as barley, rye, and oat. With this disorder, ingesting gluten causes the immune system to attack the absorptive villi in the small intestines to flatten and die,

rendering the digestion and absorption of most nutrients ineffectual. Accompanied with this damage is gastrointestinal upset, diarrhea, bloating, stomach pain, and weight loss. Left untreated, the chronic malabsorption can lead to osteoporosis, tooth decay, growth retardation in children, anemia, and fatigue. Strictly adhering to a gluten-free diet is the only effective treatment. Gluten is found in most breads, cereals, and pastas, as well as some sauces, soups, imitation meats, and even certain medications, supplements, and vitamins. There are substitutions available such as soy, rice, tapioca, corn, potato, flax seed, and buckwheat that have become increasingly popular in mainstream food products, due to the increased awareness and diagnosis of the disease in recent years. It is important for celiac patients to learn to read labels and make themselves aware of what foods contain gluten. Because many gluten-containing products are good sources of B vitamins, supplementation may be necessary for those with celiac disease.

Gastrointestinal Ulcer *tx- antacids, sucralfate + cimetidinne*

A gastrointestinal ulcer occurs when the mucosal barrier is impaired, causing the normal stomach acid entering the gastric tissue to erode the lining of the digestive tract, forming ulcers. Mucosal barrier impairment can be caused by a malfunctioning pyloric sphincter that allows acids to back up into the stomach. Causes include Helicobacter pylori (H. pylori) bacterial infections, use of NSAID drugs, emotional stress, excessive use of alcohol and cigarettes, and radiation therapy. Symptoms of gastric ulcers may include stomach discomfort, burning sensation, nausea, loss of appetite, and weight loss. To treat a gastric ulcer, antacids can be used to help neutralize acids, Cimetidine can inhibit acid secretion, and Sucralfate can help to protect the ulcer site from further damage. Nutritionally, most foods can be consumed as tolerated, although very spicy or hot foods may irritate the ulcer since they can stimulate acid secretion. Alcohol should also be limited because it can be damaging to the mucosa. Dietary intervention should focus on foods that increase patient comfort, neutralize stomach acid, and maintain a healthy gastric mucosa.

Dumping Syndrome *tx - avoid simple CHOs + refined sugars; room temp. foods. Try small meals*

Dumping syndrome commonly occurs after a patient undergoes a surgical weight loss procedure such as gastric bypass surgery, where part of the stomach is closed off or removed. After the patient returns to a normal diet, excess undigested food can build up in the jejunum because the stomach no longer has room to store food and parcel it into the intestines in smaller, timed doses. The rapid breakdown of large amounts of food can cause the intestine to become hypertonic. In an effort to restore osmotic balance, the body draws water from the plasma to dilute the large amounts of food, leading to a decrease in blood volume, sweating, weakness, rapid heartbeat, nausea, diarrhea and cramping. In addition, digested carbohydrates enter the blood, leading to elevated blood glucose, which causes an overproduction of insulin and ends in hypoglycemic conditions. For this reason, individuals at risk of dumping syndrome should limit simple carbohydrates and refined sugars, such as white breads and candy, due to the fact that they are hydrolyzed so quickly. Dairy may also need to be avoided and then slowly reintroduced as this type of food can worsen symptoms. Very hot or very cold foods can trigger symptoms and beverages should be avoided during meal times to reduce the risk of overwhelming the jejunum. Protein and healthy fats are normally well tolerated and eating small meals can help keep symptoms under control.

Diverticular Diseases *tx- Fiber intake + water*

Diverticular disease refers to three different types of conditions that can occur within the colon: diverticulosis, diverticular bleeding, and diverticulitis. Diverticulosis is the development of diverticula, which are tiny sacs or pockets along the wall of the colon. They can vary in size and tend to develop due to a very low fiber diet or loss of strength in the colon's muscle wall, leading to high pressure within the colon. Diverticula may also occur due to excessive straining of the colon during bowel movements and

Diverticulosis- sacs along intestinal wall from ↓ fiber intake (heal on its own usually)

Diverticulitis- sacs become infected/inflammed

are most common in the lower portion of the intestine, called the sigmoid colon. There may be no symptoms of diverticulosis and it is most common in the older population. Diverticular bleeding can occur due to injury or breakage of blood vessels surrounding the diverticula and resulting in large amounts of blood in stool. In most cases, this condition will heal on its own. Diverticulitis occurs when diverticula become infected or inflamed from bacteria or accumulations of fecal matter. Adhering to a diet with adequate amounts of fiber will help to prevent or ease symptoms of diverticular disease because fiber helps to ease the movement of waste through the colon, reducing pressure on the colon wall. A low residue diet may need to be followed while a patient is experiencing a diverticular flare up, after which high fiber foods can be slowly reintroduced.

Crohn's and Ulcerative Colitis

tx-hydrate + identify foods causing flare ups [handwritten]

Crohn's Large intest. [handwritten]

U.C. - rectum + lower colon [handwritten]

Crohn's disease is defined as an inflammatory disease affecting large portions of the large and small intestines. Ulcerative colitis is a similar condition but affects the rectum and lower colon. Both conditions seem to be caused by a combination of genetic, immune, bacterial and environmental factors including diets high in animal and milk proteins as well as high ratios of omega-6 to omega-3 fatty acids. Symptoms include stomach pain and upset, frequent and sudden diarrhea, blood and pus in stool, and intolerance to certain foods. Other complications such as fever, weight loss, rashes, eye inflammation, and arthritis can result. Malnutrition can become a concern due to recurrent diarrhea and self-imposed reduced food intake as a means of mitigating discomfort. With either condition, it is important to stay adequately hydrated and keep electrolyte levels within normal limits, in order to reduce flare-ups. For some patients, nutritional intervention and monitoring will be enough to manage their condition, while surgical intervention may be necessary in more severe cases. In these cases, part of the colon, and sometimes even the rectum, may be narrowed or completely removed. Rectum removal necessitates usage of a colostomy bag, to collect waste. Nutrition intervention following surgery is important because certain nutrients, specifically B vitamins, iron, and folic acid, are no longer able to be absorbed, due to the fact that the part of the colon that absorbs that vitamin has been removed. The patient will therefore need supplementation or injections. Carbohydrate and protein intake should be generous in order to restore nutritional status, following a period of time wherein nutrient intake was likely insufficient.

Diarrhea in Infants and Children

Diarrhea is a condition in which stool is excreted frequently and in a liquid form with at least three such bowel movements in one day. Due the abnormal rapidity through which the contents pass through the digestive tract with diarrhea, digestive enzymes do not have adequate time to break down the food and absorb the nutrients. Additionally, the stool passes far too quickly through the large intestine, leaving inadequate time for normal water and electrolyte reabsorption, which is why loose, watery stool is a hallmark of diarrhea. Dehydration and excessive loss of sodium and potassium can result, which is why diarrhea is particularly dangerous in infants, children, and the elderly. Signs of dehydration include irritability, loss of skin elasticity, decrease urine output, and rapid heartbeat.

Diarrhea is not a disease itself, but rather a symptom of many possible diseases, so it is important to determine the cause of the condition before trying to treat the diarrhea. It is most commonly gastroenteritis (an intestinal infection) as a result of parasite, bacteria, or virus, although there are many other causes including certain medications, lactose or food intolerances, hyperthyroidism, stress, and irritable bowel syndrome. Diarrhea is not normally dangerous and usually resolves fairly quickly. However, persistent or severe acute diarrhea can present some very serious health concerns, especially in the very young and very old. Children and infants are at a greater risk of dehydration and electrolyte imbalances, so their small bodies cannot afford to lose nutrients and fluids though frequent diarrhea. In these cases, attempts should be made to rehydrate the patient and replace fluids in the form of oral rehydration solutions, which contain sugar and salts. The World Health Organization recommends an electrolyte solution containing specific amounts of glucose, sodium, potassium, chloride, and bicarbonate in a water solution.

Steatorrhea tx- ↑ kcal intake, supplement ADEK, Ca, Fe, Mg, Zinc

Steatorrhea, a condition in which fat is not properly digested in the body and is therefore removed in the stool, can be caused by many malabsorption diseases. Normal stool contains about two to five grams of fat, whereas that of patients with steatorrhea may contain up to sixty grams of undigested fat. In order to diagnose this condition, it can be helpful to keep a food diary and collect stool samples over a period of 72 hours so that the ratio of ingested fat to excreted fat can be analyzed. Nutritional interventions will depend on the underlying cause of the condition. Patients may experience weight loss due to increased fat excretion, so increasing calorie intake can help to maintain weight. Patients may also face problems with the absorption of the fat-soluble vitamins because they rely on dietary fat for transport and absorption. In this case, it may be necessary to supplement nutrients such as calcium, iron, zinc, magnesium, and fat-soluble vitamins (A, E, D, and K).

Short Bowel Syndrome (Ileum removed - B12 supplement) Avoid ↑ fiber, sugar + fat meals

The treatment of some conditions such as cancer, Crohn's disease, ulcerative colitis, radiation therapy, or bowel obstruction may include the removal of at least half of the small intestine and all or part of the large intestine, leading to a number of issues that are collectively referred to as short bowel syndrome. Patients with short bowel syndrome have difficulties absorbing water and most nutrients, therefore malnutrition and metabolic issues such as weight loss, diarrhea, muscle wasting, dehydration, and electrolyte imbalances can result. Short bowel syndrome may also cause issues such as excessive gastric acid, increased peristalsis, and kidney or gallstone formation. Symptoms of short bowel syndrome can range in severity depending on how much of the colon was removed, which part was removed, and how well the remaining colon functions. The small intestine includes three parts: the duodenum, jejunum, and the ileum. Removal of the ileum, which is the lower portion of the small intestine, carries the additional risk of Vitamin B-12 deficiency and subsequent pernicious anemia, because this relatively small region of the digestive tract is the sole site of B-12 absorption. The patient will likely need B-12 injections every few months.

Fortunately, the remaining sections of the bowel do have the ability to adapt to a resection or removal. After such surgeries, nutrition intervention will be important for recovery and to ensure that the remaining bowel can properly adapt. In the weeks following the surgery, nutrients may need to be administered parenterally, or directly into the circulatory system. If the patient receives proper nutrition during this time, the absorptive surface of the bowel will start to increase and the patient can start to receive nutrients enterally, or directly into the stomach, duodenum, or jejunum via a feeding tube. Eventually, the patient should be able to slowly return to a normal diet, usually beginning with easily digestible liquids and working up to several small meals per day. Foods that are difficult to digest, such as those high in fat, sugar, or fiber, should be limited or avoided.

Gestational Diabetes

Gestational diabetes can occur in pregnant women, and places a strain on both the mother and the fetus. It is important to monitor the nutritional requirements of the baby, and it may be necessary for the mother to control her glucose levels with insulin therapy, even if she was previously able to control levels with diet alone. During pregnancy, insulin levels should increase. Gestational diabetes occurs when the hormones secreted by the placenta do not signal an increase in insulin production. It is important that all pregnant women be tested for gestational diabetes around 24 weeks so that nutritional intervention can take place if needed. Gestational diabetes can occur in women even if they were not diabetic before pregnancy. Normally, gestational diabetes does not affect the mother after she gives birth to the baby, although it increases her risk of developing Type 2 Diabetes. In utero, overfeeding of the fetus in diabetic mothers may occur, leading to increased birth weight. Newborn babies are at risk for hypoglycemia due to elevated insulin levels.

Gout ↓ intake of meat/fish + alcohol + ↑ water intake

Gout is a form of arthritis that occurs from increased amounts of uric acid in the blood as a result of abnormal purine metabolism. Sodium urate crystals can accumulate in the joints, tendons, and cartilage. Obesity, excessive alcohol intake, and a diet high in purines (meat and fish) are factors that can contribute to development of gout. A gouty attack most often occurs in the big toe, ankle, or knee as a sudden, sharp pain that may last for weeks or months. Generous amounts of water intake can help to alleviate pain as well as cortisone shots, and pain can diminish within a day if the patient seeks immediate treatment.

Goiters Iodine deficiency - sources shellfish, eggs, milk

A goiter is an enlargement of the thyroid gland traditionally caused by a deficiency of iodine in the diet. In the United States, iodized salts are common, so the formation of a goiter is more likely caused by the overproduction (hyperthyroidism) or underproduction (hypothyroidism) of thyroid hormones. A goiter is usually not painful, but can cause coughing and difficulty in breathing and swallowing, depending on the size of the enlargement. The RDA of iodine is 150 micrograms per day. Food sources of iodine include seafood, eggs, and milk. Goitrogens may also be present in some foods such as turnips, peanuts, and soybeans. These substances can block the absorption of iodine in the body, leading to the development of goiters. Treatment of goiters will depend on the severity of the condition as well as the underlying cause but may include nutrition therapy (with a focus on iodine consumption), surgery to remove goiter, and medications to treat inflammation, hyperthyroidism, and hypothyroidism.

Epilepsy
Epilepsy is a neurological condition that can cause chronic seizures, due to the release of excessive and disordered electrical charges. Anticonvulsant drugs may be prescribed to help prevent seizures associated with epilepsy, including phenobarbital, phenytoin, and primidone. These medications can increase the metabolism of vitamin D, so without proper vitamin D supplementation, the resultant decreased absorption of calcium can lead to osteomalacia and rickets. In some cases, moderate to severe seizures cannot be controlled with medications. A ketogenic diet may be prescribed as a last resort, as this diet is very unpalatable, causes uncomfortable side effects such as nausea and irritability, and its effects wear off after a few years. With this diet, energy needs are fulfilled mostly by fats, and nutrient supplementation is required.

Immunologic Reaction and Food Allergies
Normally, macrophages as well as T and B lymphocytes of the immune system protect the body against foreign substances, known as antigens. This is important in neutralizing proteins in the digestive system that carry the risk of causing an allergic response. There are five recognized types of antibodies, including IgG, IgM, IgD, IgA, and IgE. The IgE antibodies can bind with allergens, releasing chemicals that begin what is known as an allergic reaction. Histamine, bradykinin, and serotonin symptoms of an allergic reaction. In mild cases, symptoms include abdominal pain, coughing, hives, itching, and shortness of breath. In more severe reactions, symptoms may include shock, anaphylaxis, and even death.

Diagnostic Procedures

There are several different types of tests that can be used to diagnose food allergies. Maintaining a *diet history* as well as noting when symptoms occur can help to determine which foods lead to reactions. A family history can also help determine the causes of food allergies. A *skin prick test* is another way that food allergies can be diagnosed. This is an immunological test in which different types of food allergen are placed on the skin and a needle is used to introduce the allergen into the lower layers of the skin. The appearance of a welt measuring 3mm or larger may indicate the presence of a food allergy. This test is useful for children over age three, but younger children may not have a positive reaction even if a food allergy is present. A *double-blind food challenge* can also help diagnose food allergies. In this type of testing, a specific type of food is administered to the patient in the form of a capsule. A placebo pill is also administered. Neither the patient nor allergist knows which capsule is which until after the testing, therefore decreasing the chances of a reaction caused by anxiety or preconceptions. *Blood tests* can also be performed to test for allergies.

Dental Caries

Dental caries can also be referred to as cavities or tooth decay that destroy tooth enamel and causes cracks or pits to form on the tooth surface. They occur in the mouth when bacteria cause excess carbohydrates from the diet, specifically sucrose, to ferment and form acids, decalcifying the surface of the tooth. If left untreated, dental caries can continue to grow and destroy tooth enamel. Consumption of foods high in sugar and starches throughout the day can increase the formation of dental caries. It is less destructive to consume one large dessert as opposed to frequent snacking since acid production can continue for up to an hour after a meal. Chewing sugar-free gum can also help reduce the risk of dental caries. Diets with adequate fluoride strengthen teeth, making it more difficult for cavities to form. In some areas, a fluoride supplement may be necessary. Depending on the severity of the dental caries, treatment involves fillings, crowns, root canal surgery, or removal.

AIDS   *tx- ↑ kcal + PRO needs*

AIDS (acquired immunodeficiency syndrome) is caused by the blood-borne disease HIV (human immunodeficiency syndrome). AIDS destroys the cells of the immune system, known as T lymphocytes, which leaves the patient susceptible to opportunistic diseases such as lymphoma, Kaposi's sarcoma, and *altered brain func.* encephalopathy. The liver, kidneys, GI tract, and pancreas can be affected by complications of AIDS. Oral food intake may be painful in individuals affected by AIDS due to candidiasis. Energy needs will be increased to help fight off infections and protein malnutrition is also common. Nutrition intervention will include maintaining protein stores and preventing vitamin and mineral deficiencies that can hinder the function of the immune system.   *yeast inf.*

Eating Disorders

As mentioned, eating disorders such as anorexia and bulimia nervosa significantly affect dietary intake and put patients at risk for nutrient deficiencies and subsequent health issues. Treatment typically involves a comprehensive team approach with physicians, mental or behavioral health specialists, and experienced nutrition professionals.

Anorexia Nervosa

Anorexia Nervosa is a potentially life-threatening eating disorder in which the patient suffers from psychological issues that cause them to obsess over an ideal body image. In most cases, the individual has a distorted view of how they actually appear, leading them to starve themselves in order to lose weight. Signs that an individual is suffering from anorexia nervosa include: preoccupation with food and calories, dramatic weight loss, refusal to eat certain foods, excessive exercise, denial of hunger, and excuses to avoid meals. Symptoms of an ongoing problem with anorexia can present themselves as extreme fatigue, amenorrhea, sunken eyes and cheeks, protruding bones, weakness, fainting, inability to think clearly or concentrate, etc. Most patients suffering from anorexia will require psychological intervention in addition to nutrition interventions. It is important to reintroduce foods slowly to the patient and only when they are ready mentally and emotionally. It can help to suggest consuming small amounts of foods throughout the day, as large meals will most likely overwhelm the patient. Malnourishment is the main concern when working with a patient suffering from anorexia nervosa, so a well-balanced diet full of nutrients is crucial. In some cases, alternate methods of feeding may be necessary, such as tube feeding.

Bulimia Nervosa

Much like Anorexia nervosa, Bulimia nervosa is a serious psychological disorder that is characterized by an individual following an ongoing cycle of binge eating and purging. Purging may be accomplished by vomiting, laxatives, diuretics, or excessive exercise. Individuals suffering from this disorder have an altered sense of body image and look for extreme measures to avoid weight gain. The act of purging leads to many serious and potentially fatal health issues that can affect many systems of the body including cardiac, endocrine, and nervous systems. Purging also depletes the body of essential nutrients as well as electrolytes. Frequent vomiting may lead to damage to the digestive tract, teeth, and gums. As with anorexia, bulimia nervosa should first be treated by a mental health professional. Nutritional interventions should focus on malnourishment and slowly reintroducing a healthy, well-balanced diet.

Nutritional Screening Surveillance Systems
National surveys

- Nutrition Screening Initiative: used for the early identification of nutritional problems in the elderly. Level I screen identifies individuals who need more comprehensive assessments while the Level II screen is appropriate for potentially more serious nutritional or health issues.

- National Nutrition Monitoring and Related Research Program.

- Analyzes health and nutrition status, food consumption, and dietary attitude data from federal government agencies (USDA and DHHS).

- Pediatric Nutrition Surveillance System (HHS): assesses infant feeding practices, growth, and nutritional status, particularly in low-income, high-risk children.

- Pregnancy Nutrition Surveillance System (HHS): strives to identify and reduce pregnancy-related health risks, particularly in low-income, high-risk pregnant women. Includes factors such as maternal weight gain, anemia, breastfeeding practices, etc.

- National Health and Nutrition Examination Survey (NHANES): obtains clinical, biochemical, nutritional, and anthropometric health data on Americans. NHANES III aims to determine the nutritional issues related to aging by surveying a large sample of adults over the age of sixty-five.

- Factor Surveillance System (HHS): phone interviews regarding height, weight, smoking and alcohol usage, diabetes and other health conditions, and food frequency data for fruit and vegetable consumption.

- Youth Risk Behavior Survey (HHS): smoking and alcohol usage, weight control methods, and eating and exercise habits of high school students (grades 9 to 12).

- Weight Loss Practice Survey (HHS): gathers BMI, demographics, diet history, and self-perception data on U.S. adults currently trying to lose weight.

- USDA Nationwide Food Consumption Surveys: rates diets in U.S. households as "good" or "poor" based on the intake of seven nutrients relative to the RDA. Those that meet or exceed the RDA are "good" and those that are less than two-thirds of the RDA are rated "poor." Nutrients include vitamin A, vitamin C, protein, calcium, riboflavin, thiamin, and iron.

- Diet and Health Knowledge Survey (USDA): nutrition, food labels, and food safety knowledge questions are posed to the primary meal planner/preparer in U.S. households.

Reference Data

Reference data for National Nutrition Surveys is gathered over time and aggregated together to compare trends in the data over time. For example, since 1999, the NHANES program, one of the primary nutrition and health surveys in the United States, has been conducted annually with a shifting focus of health and nutrition topics, targeting populations to address changing needs. The surveys are disseminated to a sample group of about 5,000 different individuals each year, from various counties throughout the nation; researchers visit fifteen of these counties each year to interview random study participants. The NHANES interview process gathers demographic, socioeconomic, dietary, and health-related data. A medical examination process provided by a trained medical professional consists of medical, dental, laboratory, and physiological measurements. NHANES findings are used to assess nutrition, health status indicators, prevalence of diseases and risk factors for them, as well as form the basis for national standards or the reference data for health measurements such as weight, BMI, and blood pressure. Survey data is used in epidemiological studies and health sciences research, which are used in public health policy and to increase health knowledge and understanding in the United States. Results and statistics from prior years of the NHANES administration are available to the public on the CDC's website.

Community Health Resources Data

The CDC conducted and published the Community Health Status Indicators (CHSI) 2015, which is an online application that summarizes the health status profiles for each county in the United States in an effort to promote healthier communities through improving modifiable health factors. The profile for each county contains health indicators such as mortality and morbidity, healthcare access and quality, health behaviors, physical environment conditions, and social factors, as well as demographics. Improving social and physical environmental factors to make them more conducive to healthy work and play can improve health behaviors. County profiles and scores can be compared to others in the state and nation as well as the averages for these categories. Community food programs can include farmer's market nutrition programs, community-supported agriculture (CSA) shares, and the USDA's Commodity Supplemental Food Program (CSFP) among others.

Public Health Programs and Practices

Public health principles involve promoting aspects of a healthy diet that reduce the risk of chronic diseases. In the United States, overfeeding, obesity, and poor diet quality are the major causes of concern addressed in nutrition public policy. There are a variety of public health programs and practices that have been implemented to promote healthy living through better nutrition and physical activity. Some of these programs are available at the community- or state-level, while national programs also exist. The CDC offers online resources such as the Healthy Living webpage and the Chronic Disease Prevention and Healthy Lifestyle Promotion page, which include educational articles about nutrition as well as tools and trackers to assess disease risk, dietary intake, and physical activity. The U.S.

Department of Health and Human Services has similar resources available on their website, along with information about community resources, funding opportunities, and health statistics. Specific programs and initiatives often promote breastfeeding, the reduction of sugary beverages, increasing fruit and vegetable intake, and limiting processed foods. Menu labeling with nutrition facts and larger, easy-to-understand nutrition bullet points on beverages (such as indicating the total caloric and sugar content for the bottle and not just the serving) are examples of recently-implemented practices to improve nutrition on the population level. Legislation, such as Healthy, Hunger-Free Kids of 2010, is an example of a national initiative. Agencies such as Women, Infants, and Children (WIC) and the Le Leche League provide breastfeeding support. School meal programs, federal assistance programs such as SNAP, and nutrition PSAs are also public health programs.

Planning and Intervention

Intervention for Individuals

Interventions for individuals should be tailored to their specific needs, conditions, restrictions, and goals. In nearly all cases, the overall goal should be to improve health and prevent disease and the development of disease risk factors.

Nutrition Care for Health Promotion and Disease Prevention
Identify Desired Outcomes/Actions
The nutrition professional should identify and discuss the desired outcomes of a client's nutrition program and also consider the goals that the client may have. The developed program should be tailored to address these goals. While the variety of desired outcomes are nearly limitless, common goals for dietary plans to address include reducing body fat, overall weight, cholesterol, triglycerides, blood pressure, and blood sugar, and increasing fiber intake, protein, vegetables, and water.

Relationship of Nutrition to Maintenance of Health and Prevention of Disease
It has been well documented that diet quality can affect health and disease status. Optimal nutrition during major stages in the life cycle can help maintain health and reduce the risk of certain chronic diseases such as obesity, metabolic syndrome, diabetes, health disease, and certain cancers. Proper nutrition during infancy and childhood can reduce the risk of physical and mental growth aberrations, blindness, immune dysfunction, and behavioral and cognitive issues. Adequate nutrition during childbearing years can increase fertility and protect the mother and fetus from health conditions, such as increased risk of fracture from inadequate calcium and vitamin D intake or spina bifida from inadequate folic acid. Proper nutrition during the later stages of adulthood can help prevent sarcopenia and osteoporosis, body fat gain, and possibly even cognitive decline.

Propaganda and Popular Diets
Unfortunately, fad diets are popularized in the media daily. The weight-loss industry is a multi-billion-dollar industry for a reason: people are desperate to lose weight and are often looking for a "quick, easy fix," which many of these diets and exercise gadgets promise. However, many of these fad diets are dangerous or not developed by consummate professionals with any scientific research to validate their safety or efficacy, eliminating entire food groups or claiming the diet to be some sort of health panacea. Other unhealthy methods promising rapid weight loss in popular culture include exercising in saunas or steam rooms to "sweat off pounds," starvation or liquid diets, cleanses, and mega dosing dietary supplements. These can cause dangerous dehydration, overdose on certain supplements, electrolyte imbalances that can cause arrhythmias, and loss of resting metabolic rate when the body senses starvation, making subsequent weight loss harder. Nutrition professionals should be aware that clients

may inquire about such diets and fitness gadgets. When they do, nutrition experts should remember that it may take patience as well as targeted and thorough education to convey the danger and ineffectiveness of such methods and provide the alternative realities for healthy weight loss.

Determining Energy/Nutrient Needs Specific to Life Span Stage

While all humans need the same types of macro- and micronutrients, specific needs vary according to life span stage. Dietary Reference Intakes (DRIs) are published for healthy individuals at each life stage. It should be noted that diets high in whole grains, vegetables, lean proteins, and legumes are recommended for all ages to reduce the risk of various diseases. Energy, macronutrient, and micronutrient needs are highest in young children relative to body size. Specific nutrient needs, such as folic acid and calcium, are higher for pregnant and lactating mothers than at other life stages, and the needs for elderly adults are such that certain nutrient requirements increase (such as vitamin D), while total caloric intake and other specific nutrients (like iron) decrease.

Menu Planning for Health Promotion

After a comprehensive intake process, in which the nutrition professional learns about the health conditions, current dietary practices, nutritional needs, food preferences, cultural factors, economic and food access factors, and goals of the client, a meal plan is developed tailored to the client. Menu planning for health promotion is one of the most important tasks of a nutrition professional. Plans must provide adequate nutrition for the specific client, as well as be practical and agreeable to that client.

Nutritional Adequacy

First and foremost, menu planning for health promotion must consider the nutritional requirements of the client and be designed to meet those needs. As mentioned, many factors affect the nutrient requirements for a given client, including age, sex, health status, body size, and activity level.

Client Acceptance, Diet Patterns, Schedules

Menu plans must be compatible with the client's diet pattern and eating schedule. While it may be ideal from a health standpoint for a specific client to eat five or six smaller meals per day, if his or her schedule is such that there is only ample time to eat two or three times daily, the nutrition professional needs to find a way to meet the same dietary goals within these confines. It is prudent to suggest the optimal plan include the frequency and timing of meals, and then discuss its feasibility with the client. Certain diet patterns may be modifiable.

Socio-Cultural Ethnic Factors

Socio-cultural ethnic factors can affect food preferences, diet patterns, and eating schedules. Nutrition professionals need to be sensitive and respectful of cultural food practices and find ways to modify "ideal" plans so that they work within the ethnic ideals or rituals of the client's cultural identity. Certain cultures avoid food groups or products all together (such as dairy, or specific proteins), while others place significance or frequent reliance on unhealthy foods, such as fried food, high-fat proteins, and sweets, and limit the intake of desirable options, such as vegetables. It should be noted that food is a central part of the celebrations and gatherings in most cultures, and many people have strong emotional ties to food choices and rituals. When possible, nutrition professionals can suggest ways to modify or substitute less healthy options for more ideal selections.

Substitutions and Food Preferences

The most successful meal plans are the ones that clients follow. While menu planning should meet nutritional needs, the diet's ability to improve health is contingent upon it being followed. As such, it is crucial that nutritional professionals obtain a comprehensive understanding of a client's food preferences during intake. These foods should not be included on the client's menu plan. Where possible, substitutions should be suggested, particularly in cases where the client expresses flexibility and openness to explore other options. In such cases, nutrition professionals should not only explain how and what to substitute but educate clients on why such substitution is important and beneficial. Arming clients with knowledge can increase their motivation and willingness to improve their diet. It is sometimes prudent to make substitutions in gradual steps, as this approach can be more acceptable and comfortable for the client. For example, for a client eating fried chicken from a local fast food chain every day at lunch, suggesting a spinach salad with baked salmon, egg, tomatoes, and other fresh vegetables can be an overwhelming and unappealing switch. Instead, smaller swaps can be implemented in a step-wise manner over a couple weeks. Perhaps first buying a salad at the fast food place along with the regular meal can begin the movement in the right direction in a manageable way.

Cost Factors

Factors related to cost can significantly impact dietary intake and must be considered in successful menu planning; if a client or dietary center cannot afford the suggested menu or food plan, it will be of no use. Unfortunately, the reality in the United States is that many of the healthiest food choices, especially organic foods, are more expensive than unhealthy options. This further incentivizes consumers to select cheaper and easier options like fast food and highly processed choices. Nutrition professionals should learn and teach cost-saving strategies such as buying in bulk, selecting frozen vegetables over fresh when necessary, choosing store-brand options, using coupons, shopping sales, selecting less expensive healthy alternatives (such as beans and brown rice or less expensive cuts of meat and how to prepare them), and advising those food items that should be purchased organic, if possible (such as produce with thin skins on the "Dirty Dozen" list). While conversations about finances are inherently somewhat uncomfortable, it is important that menus fall within the client's food budget.

Food Labeling

An integral component of successful meal planning and dietary improvements for clients is educating them on how to read and interpret food labels. Food products produced in the United States must adhere to labeling requirements, including listing all ingredients and additives. This information can inform consumers about the profile of the product prior to consumption. Clients should be advised to avoid foods with chemical additives and preservatives whenever possible, those with unhealthy nutrition profiles, and those with unhealthy ingredients (such as hydrogenated oils, refined sugars and grains, or artificial food products) leading off the ingredient list.

Recipe Modification

Recipe modification involves identifying and implementing changes or substitutions to the ingredients and/or preparation methods of recipes to improve their nutrient profile. This strategy is particularly helpful for clients with strong attachments to various meals, either for cultural, social, emotional, or practical reasons, but for whom those meals, as is, are unhealthy. Modifications may include changes such as reducing added salt or oil, baking or roasting instead of frying or sautéing, adding vegetables, reducing the proportion of starches or added fats, overall portion adjustments, and substituting in whole grain options or leaner proteins in place of refined grains or lower-quality proteins.

Culinary Demonstrations

Culinary demonstrations can be offered in public community settings, grocery stores, private classes, television, and other media. While these can have an array of purposes, some are aimed at teaching individuals what and how to cook healthy meals at home. Lack of knowledge regarding menu planning and food preparation can increase the reliance on unhealthy fast food or frozen and prepared foods.

Nutrition professionals can either conduct or suggest healthy culinary demonstrations to educate new home cooks or those who need modification to their food preparation routines.

Grocery Store Tours

Grocery store tours are an increasingly popular educational tactic in the nutrition field. Nutrition professionals can take individual clients or community groups into local grocery stores and markets and essentially do a shopping walk-through, in which the nutrition expert educates shoppers on smart and healthy purchases. He or she may advise consumers on how to select produce to maximize health benefits and minimize cost (such as buying in-season fruits and vegetables or those that are flash-frozen, which preserves their nutrient content), how to identify healthier choices and substitutions, where to find the most nutrient-dense options, and how to find and use sales and coupons to save money.

Medical Nutrition Therapy and Planning

Medical Nutrition Therapy (MNT) is the implementation of a specifically tailored dietary plan to address a client's medical condition and its associated symptoms. These diets are developed in collaboration with medical professionals, using the patient's medical record, physical exam data, symptoms and limitations, and physical presentation. The goal of MNT is to ameliorate the symptoms or disease effects and prevent exacerbation of the disease or health condition. MNT is frequently used for those with type 2 diabetes, high cholesterol, or receiving dialysis.

Treatment of Major-Related Disorders or Conditions start

Cardiovascular

Heart Disease ↑↑ - LS|LF

Cardiovascular disease is a very common disease that can be easily prevented, in most cases, by following a healthy diet and lifestyle. Patients who have already developed heart problems can suffer from complications such as high blood pressure, blocked blood vessels, high risk of heart attack or stroke. Developing and following a healthy diet can help to decrease these risks. Generally, patients with cardiovascular disease will want to follow a low sodium, low cholesterol, and low-fat diet. Patients should aim for less than 2300 mg (about 1 teaspoon) of sodium per day, and less than 300 mg of cholesterol per day. Foods that are high in trans fats such as fried foods, packaged baked goods, and processed foods should be avoided due to the fact that too much trans-fat can raise LDL cholesterol levels in the blood. Increasing the amount of fruit, vegetables, and healthy whole grains in the diet can help heart disease patients decrease their risk of complications. They are high in essential vitamins and minerals and may aid in weight loss, which will reduce symptoms and risks.

Congestive Heart Failure - LS ⊕ diuretics("waterpills")to promote urine output from edema

Congestive heart failure occurs gradually over a period of time as the heart slowly loses its ability to function properly. In the early stages of the disease, the heart begins to enlarge, and heart rate increases. Eventually, patients may experience symptoms such as shortness of breath, chest pain, and changes in blood pressure, due to impairment of normal blood circulation. This can lead to the reabsorption of sodium and resultant edema in the legs, and because of this swelling, anthropometric measurements can be inaccurate and not an ideal means of assessment. Decreased circulation allows sodium and fluid to accumulate in tissues, so a low sodium diet and diuretics may be recommended to help prevent further damage to the heart and improve edema. However, since diuretics can deplete potassium, a potassium supplement may be needed.

Hypertension ~~tx~~ - LS + diuretics ⊕ K supplementation

Hypertension is defined as a systolic blood pressure of 140 or higher and a diastolic blood pressure of 90 or higher. There are a number of different physiologic systems that contribute to blood pressure levels, including the volume of fluid in the vascular system, strength of heart contractions and muscular walls of the arterioles, and vessel diameter. The kidneys, heart, and nervous system work to maintain normal blood pressure levels. Specifically, excess sodium that cannot be excreted by the kidney can lead to increased levels of sodium and water in the blood, causing an elevated plasma volume. This increase in interstitial sodium may also increase calcium levels in vessel musculature, leading to rigidity, and further elevating blood pressure. In obese patients, higher insulin levels can cause the kidneys to reabsorb sodium, putting these individuals at a greater risk of hypertension.

Managing Hypertension Through Medication and Diet

Diuretics and antihypertensive medications are typically prescribed to treat hypertension. Although diuretics help to decrease fluid volume and sodium levels in the body, they can decrease potassium levels (hypokalemia), so an increase in dietary potassium or a potassium-sparring medication can be helpful. Other treatments for hypertension include weight loss, low sodium diets, decreased alcohol intake, and increased exercise. The sodium recommendation for patients with hypertension is 1500 mg/day or less. Alcohol intake should be limited to less than three drinks per day.

Critical Care

usually:
(35-45 kcal/kg, 30% Fat, 1-2 g/kg) ← PRO

Injury Recovery

In accident victims, nutritional intervention should begin as soon as the patient is back to a stable condition. Protein loss, nitrogen balance, and loss of lean body tissue are the most critical issues that should be addressed following trauma. Protein loss can lead to complications such as hypoalbuminemia, infections, slow wound healing, breakdown of skin, and decreased function of the immune system. Nitrogen balance may not be achieved within the first few days, but loss of lean body tissue can be prevented. In the days following an injury, enteral feeding may be necessary. The severity of the injury will determine the carbohydrate and protein needs of the patient. In most cases, the patient's needs will be satisfied by 35 to 45 kcal/kg. Lipids should provide about 30 percent of calories. Protein needs will range from 1 to 2 g/kg, depending on severity of trauma. Oral feeding should be delayed for 24 to 48 hours following surgery in order for normal peristalsis activity to return. Fluid and electrolyte balance should be closely monitored post-surgery in order to ensure that balance is returning to normal and may need to be administered intravenously.

Burns

Extensive burns can lead to an increase in basal energy expenditure by 100 percent or more. Significant protein, fluid, and electrolytes are lost through the wound, so intake of all three must increase. Increased energy intake is required to meet the needs of wound healing and fighting off the possibility of infection. Recommendations of caloric intake can be determined by implementing a formula that considers body weight as well as the total body surface area that has been burned. Protein needs are increased in burn patients in order to maintain nitrogen balance and help in wound healing because severe burns increase protein catabolism and nitrogen excretion. In addition, supplementation with vitamin C, magnesium, and zinc is helpful, especially in patients receiving parenteral nutrition or patients who may already have a zinc deficiency. Vitamin C is helpful in collagen formation and therefore crucial to the wound healing process. Magnesium is lost in significant amounts from the wounds, and zinc also aids in the wound healing process.

Metabolic Disorders

Diabetes

Diabetes is defined as a disease in which the pancreas either does not produce insulin (Type 1) or the body is not receptive to the insulin in circulation (Type 2). Insulin is a hormone that is used in the body to regulate the amount of glucose in the blood stream. When carbohydrates are consumed, they are broken down in the body and converted to glucose, or blood sugar. It is the job of insulin to promote the uptake of glucose by the cells, particularly muscle and liver cells. In a patient with Type 1 or Type 2 diabetes, this system is not functioning properly or not at all, causing glucose to remain in the bloodstream, which leads to hyperglycemia, or high blood sugar. This, in turn, prevents the cells from receiving the glucose they require for energy. Some common, general symptoms of Diabetes include fatigue, increased thirst and increased hunger, frequent urination, dry mouth and skin, and blurry vision. Patients with diabetes can live long and healthy lives if their condition is properly managed. If it is not, risk of complications such as blindness, stroke, circulation issues in extremities, and heart disease are increased.

Type 1 Diabetes

Type 1 diabetes is a rarer form of diabetes (about 5 to 10 percent of cases) and is usually diagnosed early in life. This type may also be referred to as juvenile-onset or insulin dependent diabetes. It occurs when the body does not produce insulin at all. It is thought that Type 1 diabetes is caused by genetics. People living with this disease must administer insulin via a subcutaneous injection or an insulin pump in order to assure their body is receiving the hormone.

Type 2 Diabetes

Type 2 diabetes is a more common form of diabetes and usually develops more gradually throughout life. People with this type do produce insulin, but it does not perform its proper function of providing fuel to the cells. Therefore, it may also be referred to as insulin-resistant diabetes. Type 2 is thought to be caused by poor diet and lifestyle habits.

How Diabetes May Affect One's Dietary Needs

Following a proper diet is extremely important for patients with diabetes. It is particularly crucial for diabetics to monitor their intake of carbohydrates, due to the fact that they are converted to glucose, or sugar in the body. Since the basis of diabetes is the process of breaking down carbohydrates into glucose and its subsequent absorption into the cells for fuel, attention must be given to carbohydrate intake. A well-balanced diet according to the MyPlate guidelines should be followed, but many nutrition professionals recommend utilizing a carbohydrate exchange diet. An exchange diet is a method of allowing the patient to still enjoy a well-rounded diet, but closely monitoring starch intake, known as "counting carbs." Patients will use the Diabetic Exchange List to make food choices that will help them to keep daily starch intake at a reasonable amount. This list groups foods together that are similar in their carbohydrate, protein, fat, and calorie content. This allows the patient to interchange foods from the same list to add variety to the diet. Sugar-free or artificially sweetened products are satisfactory choices for diabetic patients, as these do not have an effect on blood glucose levels. Patients should also avoid foods high in saturated fats, cholesterol, and sodium, as they are already at an increased risk of heart disease.

Recommendations for Protein, Fat, and Carbohydrate Intake

There is no evidence that suggests that protein intake needs to be adjusted for a diabetic patient. They should follow the same guidelines as the general population, which is 15 to 20 percent of the total daily energy intake, or 0.8g/kg for adults and 1 to 2.2g/kg for children. Dietary fat intake is also similar to the general population, but should be carefully monitored in diabetic patients, as a diet low in trans- and saturated fats can help decrease LDL cholesterol. This is important for everyone, but especially diabetics, as they are already at an increased risk of heart disease. As a general rule, total fat intake should account for less than 30 percent of the total daily intake and saturated fat should make up less than 10 percent. As stated earlier, carbohydrate intake must be closely monitored in diabetic patients. The recommended daily intake will vary from patient to patient depending on their individual blood glucose responses, but will normally range from 55 to 60 percent of the daily total energy intake.

start ↓ Obesity

The Body Mass Index measurement (BMI=weight in kilograms/height in meters^2) is a method of determining whether an individual is at a healthy weight, underweight, overweight, or obese. Based on a predetermined chart, an individual with a BMI of 25.1 to 30 is considered overweight, and a BMI of 30.1 to 40 is considered obese. Obesity can be caused by a variety of factors including environment, culture, heredity, and psychological issues. Genetically, factors such as resting metabolic rate, size and number of fat cells, and hormonal and neurological influences that control satiety can lead to obesity. It is theorized that individuals are born with a predetermined weight, which is controls by fat stores in the body. Regardless of lifestyle, eating, and exercise habits, an individual will eventually return to this weight in order to maintain a homeostatic balance, according to this theory. Obesity is a major risk factor that can contribute to many more serious diseases and complications, including diabetes, heart disease, arthritis, high blood pressure, stroke, breathing difficulties, gallstones, and some cancers.

Nutritional Care

Nutritional intervention of obese patients is similar to the treatment of a chronic illness, since the patient will need ongoing monitoring in order to maintain their weight. It can be very difficult for obese patients to keep the weight off after they have lost a significant amount, especially if it was lost quickly, resulting in a process known as weight cycling. In some cases, a patient will regain more weight than was originally lost, and in even higher percentages of adipose tissue. This process of gaining and losing weight can lead to metabolic issues. In other cases, an individual will reach a "plateau," where weight loss dramatically slows or stops completely. It is important to focus on healthy eating, exercise, and behavior changes in order to be successful in a weight loss program. All of these aspects should lead to a steady weight loss over time, decreasing the chance that the individual will regain the weight or hit a plateau. A slower weight loss also helps to reduce fat stores while preserving lean body tissues, which can maintain metabolic rate.

Gastrointestinal

Hepatic

Cirrhosis of the liver is a disease that progresses slowly. It occurs when healthy liver tissue is replaced with scar tissue, which segments it with fibrous bands and inhibits proper hepatic blood flow and nutrient processing. Causes of liver cirrhosis can include hepatitis, cystic fibrosis, fatty liver disease, diabetes, and alcoholism. The portal vein is a large vessel that carries blood to the liver. Limited blood circulation causes increased pressure to the portal vein, leading to other veins within the circulatory system to enlarge and bypass the liver. This can then lead to an increased risk of hemorrhaging and a backup of fluid into the peritoneal cavity. Because of the liver's central role in detoxification, when the liver function is compromised, toxins remain in the bloodstream and are carried to the brain, causing confusion, behavioral changes, and even coma.

Consumption of alcohol can have different effects on the body, depending on the amount. Because alcohol provides 7 kcal/g but no other vitamins, minerals, protein, or fat, light drinking causes minimal disturbance to nutrient intake, provided that the individual is also consuming a healthy diet. On the other hand, individuals who drink heavily may be replacing significant amounts of food with alcohol, therefore missing out on essential nutrients the body needs to function. Triglycerides are deposited in the liver after alcohol is metabolized, which can cause fatty liver over time. Risk of hypoglycemia is increased due to the disruption of pyruvate metabolism and glycogen storage. Inflammation of the stomach, pancreas, and intestines due to heavy alcohol consumption decreases the absorption of vitamin C, vitamin B-12, thiamin, and folic acid, depressing immune, cognitive, and cardiac function. Thiamin deficiency can lead to dementia. In addition, alcohol is metabolized to acetaldehyde, leading to hepatic toxicity, which impairs the liver's ability to utilize vitamins A, D, B-6, and folic acid. An alcoholic has an increased need for various B complex vitamins, which worsens the problem of vitamin B impairment.

Nutritional Management
Eventually, cirrhosis of the liver may lead to complete liver failure, which is defined as the liver's function being reduced to 30 percent or less. Since the liver will no longer be able to properly metabolize fat, caloric intake of fat should be reduced to 25 percent. Long chain fatty acids are difficult to digest, so they can be replaced by medium-chained triglycerides, such as those found in coconut oil. In this case, linoleic acid supplementation may be necessary to avoid the development of essential fatty acid deficiency. Due to lack of bile salts, pancreatic insufficiency, or portal vein blockage, fat may be present in the stool of patients suffering from cirrhosis. In this case, supplementation of vitamin A, D, E, and K (fat soluble vitamins) may be necessary. As mentioned, thiamin and Vitamin B-12 deficiencies may also require supplementation. Risk of hepatic encephalopathy is increased due to an imbalance of branched-chain amino acids (BCAA) and altered protein metabolism. Neomycin may be used in an attempt to reduce blood ammonia, and lactulose may be used to induce diarrhea and remove contents from the intestine. Sodium restriction (500 to 2000 mg/day) and diuretics can help manage fluid accumulation in the peritoneal cavity, known as ascites.

Gallbladder
The function of the gallbladder is to store and concentrate bile that has been secreted by the liver. The sphincter of Oddi is relaxed after food is ingested and bile is released via the common bile duct into the duodenum. Water and electrolytes are absorbed by the mucosa, creating a product containing high concentrations of bile salt and cholesterol. Bile is important in the absorption of fats, fat-soluble vitamins, calcium, and iron. The gallbladder is prone to diseases such as gallstones (cholelithiasis) and inflammation (cholecystitis). Gallstones occur when stones slip into the common bile duct, leading to cramping. Inflammation is a result of gallstones blocking the opening of the duct, causing backup of bile into the gallbladder and possible infection.

Surgical intervention is the typical treatment of gallbladder issues. In most cases, the gallbladder is removed completely, therefore shifting the job of bile storage into the common duct between the liver and small intestine. The first few days following a surgical procedure, enteral feeding may be necessary. The patient can then return to a normal diet but should limit fat intake for the first month, so that the inflammation can resolve. If surgery is not an option for the patient, a low fat diet (about 25 percent kcals) should be followed, and supplementation with fat-soluble vitamins is necessary.

Pancreatic
The pancreas is both an endocrine and exocrine organ and has functions in the digestive and endocrine systems. Endocrine cells are important in the production of insulin and glucagon and exocrine cells help to digest carbohydrates, fats, and proteins in the chyme. Pancreatitis, or inflammation of the pancreas, involves pus accumulation, fat necrosis, and edema, and can often be caused by recurrent gallstones and excessive alcohol consumption. Symptoms can range in severity but can include severe stomach

pain that radiates to the back, jaundice, pale stool, dark urine, and shock. Because the pancreatic exocrine enzymes such as amylase and lipase can damage the structures of the pancreas and surrounding organs, early detection via serum amylase levels, fat in stool, and glucose tolerance is important.

Nutritional Management

Ingestion of food can cause an exacerbation of painful pancreatitis symptoms. Parenteral nutrition directly into the patient's circulatory system may be necessary if normal eating is too painful. Some patients may tolerate clear liquid diets or several small meals throughout the day, although it is imperative that such meals are very low in fat and do not include any alcohol. Eventually, replacement of pancreatic enzymes may be necessary due to complete loss of pancreatic function.

Malnutrition

Malnutrition is a general term referring to the condition resulting from consuming a diet with insufficient or excessive nutrients such that health problems ensue. Malnutrition can involve one or all of the following nutrient categories: total caloric intake, specific macronutrients—mainly carbohydrates or protein—and micronutrients (vitamins or minerals). Undernutrition (insufficient nutrient intake) during pregnancy, infancy, or childhood can result in permanent physical and mental developmental issues. Specific short- and long-term health consequences of malnutrition depend on the specific nutrition issue but can include general starvation, shortened statute, poor immunity, poor muscle tone, swollen abdomen, unhealthy body composition, and issues with vision, cognition, and disease status. Poverty and high food prices are the main causes of underfeeding.

Protein-Calorie

Although malnutrition can refer to either overfeeding or underfeeding conditions, it typically refers to undernourishment, particularly with protein and energy, wherein a cellular imbalance exists between the body's demand for protein and energy for growth, maintenance, function, and the supply (intake). Protein-Energy Malnutrition (PEM) can result in wasting (excessively low weight for height) or stunting (reduced stature or inability to reach growth potential). The most common risk factors for PEM include lack of high quality or total food, gastrointestinal illnesses such as parasites, conditions leading to malabsorption, chronic illnesses, and poor sanitation. Stunting and wasting are particularly prevalent in the "developing world," where about one-third of children suffer from one or both conditions due to PEM. PEM falls into one of two distinct disorders: marasmus and kwashiorkor. Marasmus is a wasting disease, which results from an inadequate caloric and protein intake. There is severe wasting, very little body fat, muscle wasting, and very little swelling. It occurs in cases of prolonged famine or starvation, and severe cases of anorexia nervosa. Kwashiorkor is predominated by a lack of sufficient protein. The body tends to swell, with edema particularly concentrated in the extremities and abdomen. Some wasting may also occur, along with liver enlargement, loss of skin and hair pigmentation, and hypoalbuminaemia. It should be noted that micronutrient deficiencies are present in nearly all cases of PEM.

Vitamin

Vitamin malnutrition falls under the umbrella of micronutrient malnutrition. Micronutrient malnutrition can be concurrent with PEM or macronutrient deficiencies, but can also occur in isolation, wherein specific vitamins and minerals are deficient. In those with PEM, micronutrient deficiencies are nearly inevitable, because the entire quantity and quality of the diet is inadequate. The etiology of specific micronutrient deficiencies in isolation or combinations can be more complicated. The following list contains some of the more common vitamin deficiencies, their causes, and symptoms:

Vitamin A Deficiency - blindness

Deficiencies in vitamin A are infrequent in "developed" countries but occur frequently in "developing" nations, and such deficiency is the leading cause of preventable blindness. It also results in poor immunity, dry skin and hair, impaired bone growth, and increased risk for infections.

Vitamin B

Vitamin B is a complex of roughly a dozen identified vitamins and deficiencies that can occur in one, multiple, or all of the included vitamins. The most common vitamin B deficiency worldwide is usually cited to be B12. Because this vitamin is bacteria that occurs in dirt and water, it is found mostly in animal products (animals that graze dirt and drink unfiltered water). Individuals following vegan diets or with limited access to animal products, as well as those with impaired absorption (those lacking intrinsic factor) or with diseases of malabsorption (such as H. pylori-induced chronic gastritis or bacterial overgrowth) are most susceptible to a Vitamin B12 deficiency. While most people are asymptomatic, symptoms of deficiency can include decreased mental capacity and memory, decreased proprioception, weakness and numbness in the extremities, poor coordination, and impaired sense of smell, among others. Vitamin B3 or niacin deficiency (frequently in concert with deficiencies in other micronutrients or amino acids) can result in pellagra. Such a deficiency is most common in corn-dominant diets, as well as in individuals in South Asia who consume a significant amount of millet, which has a high leucine content. Symptoms include a butterfly-shaped facial rash, diarrhea, anxiety, and tremors. Vitamin B1 or thiamine deficiency can lead to beriberi, which refers to a group of symptoms including peripheral neuropathy, weakness, appetite loss, constipation, and heart failure. This deficiency is most common in those whose diets are of poor quality, composed of mostly white rice, alcoholics, those with chronic liver or thyroid disease, those with chronic diarrhea, and breastfeeding or pregnant individuals consuming a poor diet.

Vitamin C

Deficiencies in vitamin C in "developed" countries result from states of chronic malnutrition or absorption, chronic diarrhea, alcoholism, and diets devoid of vegetables and fruit. The symptoms manifest as scurvy and occur because vitamin C is crucial for collagen synthesis; in the absence of a sufficient amount, individuals can experience bleeding gums, poor wound healing, ecchymosis, weakness, fatigue, edema, depression, and neuropathy, among others.

Vitamin D

High rates of deficiency have been observed in both "developed" and "developing" countries, often in combination with inadequate dietary intake of calcium and iron. However, because a significant portion of vitamin D absorption is transdermal, inadequacy often is due to factors outside of diet including limited sun exposure from clothing, lifestyle, or environment; dark skin tone/pigment; reduced capacity for vitamin D synthesis (a product of aging and some medical conditions); diseases of malabsorption like celiac; and in pregnant or lactating mothers and their infants. Vitamin D deficiency can lead to rickets, osteoporosis, and hormonal issues.

Mineral

The most common mineral deficiencies and their resultant symptoms are as follows:

Iron

The most common nutritional deficiency on a global scale is iron deficiency. In fact, it is estimated to affect 50 percent of children living in "developing" nationals, particularly infants, young children, and women of childbearing age. Risk increases in babies that continue to breastfeed after six months of age without iron supplementation or who do wean, but with only low-iron foods. Insufficient bioavailability of dietary iron can result in iron-deficiency anemia, and is more common in diets that inhibit the absorption of iron, such as those with high levels of tannins in tea and phytates from certain plants. The condition can also result from parasitic infections such as hookworm or malaria, and hemoglobinopathies, including sickle cell disease, thalassemia, and chronic infections. During periods of rapid growth (between 6 to 24 months), chronic iron deficiency is associated with impaired psychomotor and cognitive development. In adults, it reduces energy and reproductive function.

Zinc

Because zinc plays an integral role in growth and development as it is required for the catalytic activity for dozens of enzymes, deficiency can cause growth retardation and delayed sexual maturation, appetite loss, diarrhea, and impaired wound healing and immune function.

Iodine

Iodine deficiency is estimated to affect slightly more than 30 percent of school-aged children. Iodine is an essential component of thyroid hormones, so deficiency is the leading cause of thyroid disease, as well as physical and mental retardation, goiter, and other growth and developmental abnormalities. Iodine is a trace mineral found in soil and seafood, and the implementation of universal salt iodization has helped reduce the prevalence of deficiency.

Cancer

Cancer is a disease where there is abnormal cell growth, which can spread throughout the body. Cancer treatments can cause a number of side effects including fatigue, altered sense of taste and smell, nausea, and dry mouth. Cancer patients have a weakened immune system, so it is important to ensure that they follow a diet with adequate amounts of vitamins and minerals. For this reason, any food with the potential to carry bacteria should be avoided, such as raw or undercooked meats. Proper food safety and sanitation techniques will become even more crucial. Because cancer patients frequently suffer from fatigue, increasing calorie intake to promote energy may be beneficial. Cancer can cause patients to experience a loss of appetite due to changes in their sense of taste. Foods may begin to taste metallic or bland, so it is important to offer methods to combat these issues, such as flavoring beverages, using herbs and spices, or using gum and mints. Depending on the type of cancer, mouth sores, esophageal issues, or gum disease can make consuming regular foods uncomfortable. In this case, tube feeding or liquid diets may need to be used.

Chemotherapy

Chemotherapy cancer treatments kill rapidly dividing cells, so complications of the GI tract such as nausea, vomiting, diarrhea, mouth sores, and inflammation of the esophagus can result. Nutritional intervention should address these issues as well as the taste aversions that arise due to metallic tasting foods and altered sense of smell. Meat is commonly not well tolerated in patients receiving chemotherapy, so protein may need to come from sources such as soy, cottage cheese, and other bland dairy foods. Serving foods cold or at room temperature can improve palatability, but enteral or parenteral feeding may be necessary if GI function is lost.

Renal Disorders   *Avoid multi-vitamins, LS, Ca supplement*

Kidney Disease is defined as the condition in which the kidneys cannot eliminate waste and fluid from the body and blood. This leads to a buildup of fluids, causing swelling in the ankles and feet, known as edema, nausea, weakness, and increased blood pressure. If kidney disease is not treated in a timely manner, the condition can worsen and potentially be fatal.

The function of a healthy kidney is to filter and eliminate waste after the body has digested food, after muscle activity, and after ingesting medications. The kidneys are also responsible for sustaining a proper balance of water and minerals, particularly sodium, phosphorus, and potassium in the blood stream.

They are important for the production of Vitamin D and red blood cells. Once kidneys fail completely, a patient will undergo dialysis treatments in order to restore blood to a healthy state and replace the job of the kidneys. This treatment uses a special machine to filter and remove wastes and excess fluid from the body.

Before a patient reaches the level of complete kidney failure and requires dialysis, there are nutritional interventions that must be utilized. Specifically, protein, sodium, potassium, phosphorus, and calcium should be monitored. When kidneys are not working correctly, they cannot handle a significant amount of protein, so it is important to limit protein intake while still getting enough to maintain body function. The patient's diet must include the right balance of healthy protein sources, as well as carbohydrates and fat that the body can use for energy. Consuming enough carbohydrates and fat will allow the body to utilize the protein to repair cells. Sodium intake must be carefully monitored and consumption should be limited. Patients with kidney disease already have trouble moving and eliminating fluids from the body, and sodium can cause the body to retain even more fluids. This leads to complications such as high blood pressure. Potassium and phosphorus levels in the body can increase in a patient with kidney disease, which can affect the heart, so it may be important to limit intake of this mineral. When phosphorus levels increase, it can cause calcium levels to decrease, so a patient with kidney disease may need to increase calcium in their diet, either by food sources or a supplement. Patients should also avoid taking multivitamins, as their body already has a hard time breaking down nutrients, and this makes it more difficult to maintain the proper balance of vitamins and minerals.

Respiratory Disorders

COPD   ↑ kcal, ↓ LS ↓ ↓ fluids, may need diruetics

COPD, chronic obstructive pulmonary disease, is an obstruction of the airway that develops from chronic bronchitis, emphysema, or asthma. Chronic bronchitis is defined as a severe, productive cough that does not resolve. Emphysema is a condition in which the air sacs (alveoli) become enlarged, walls are degraded, and elasticity is lost. Severe COPD can lead to heart problems due to increased pressure on the pulmonary arteries, called cor pulmonale. The goal of nutritional intervention should be to prevent malnourishment, which is a risk for COPD patients due to increased energy needs as well as increased oxygen consumption. Edema is also common in individuals with COPD, which can mask weight loss, due to swelling. For this reason, weight should be closely monitored. Restricting sodium and fluids can help most patients with edema, but diuretics may be necessary in some cases. Energy requirements are increased so high calorie liquid supplements may be helpful.

Cystic Fibrosis   ↑ Na ↑ ↑ kcal

Cystic fibrosis, a genetic disease, affects lung, pancreas, liver, kidney, and intestine function. Thick secretions, with the consistency of mucous, block airways and ducts and prevent the pancreas from releasing digestive enzymes, leading to malabsorption of major nutrients. Other symptoms include shortness of breath, coughing, infections, and impaired sense of smell, which can lead to poor food intake. Due to malabsorption, enzyme replacement therapy may be necessary and calorie intake should be increased to 120 percent to 150 percent RDA. Due to increased amounts lost in sweat, sodium intake should be increased as well. Since fat is not properly absorbed in patients with cystic fibrosis, supplementation of fat-soluble vitamins may be necessary. Diabetes can eventually occur due to damage of the pancreas over time.

Acute Respiratory Distress Syndrome   ↑ PRO ↑ Fat, ↓ CHO

Patients with chronic obstructive pulmonary disease may experience acute respiratory failure when the respiratory muscles become too weak for the lungs to maintain blood oxygen at a sufficient functional level via gas exchange. In most cases, patients already have a poor nutritional status, which may worsen during a hospital stay. Goals of nutritional intervention include preservation of lean body mass, prevention of further weight loss, and maintenance of fluid balance. Protein should be increased so that patients have a greater chance of weaning off of mechanical ventilation. Because carbohydrate intake can increase carbon dioxide production, intake should be restricted and half of all non-protein calories should come from fat instead. If the patient's digestive system is functioning, enteral feeding may be recommended, but care should be taken in tube placement to avoid aspiration.

Wound Care

Pressure Ulcers ↑ protein needs + well-balanced diet

A pressure ulcer is an area of the skin that is broken down due to prolonged rubbing or pressure. This condition may also be referred to as bedsores, decubitus ulcers, or pressure sores. A pressure ulcer occurs when the outer layer of skin is worn down overtime and can reach as deep as the muscle, bone, tendons, and other tissues. An ulcer can be the result of immobility (such as in bedridden or wheelchair-bound patients), incontinence (moisture can worsen the development of sores), diabetes, or circulation problems. The appearance of pressure ulcers can be a sign of malnourishment, so it is important for affected individuals to follow a healthy, well balanced diet. An increase in protein intake may benefit the patient and help them to heal more quickly.

Determination of Energy/Nutrient Needs Specific to Condition
Energy and nutrient needs are met through the consumption of fluids, macronutrients (fats, carbohydrates, and proteins), and vitamin and mineral supplements. Energy and nutrient needs will vary based on individual factors such as basal metabolic rate, sex, age, body composition, health status, health and fitness goals, physical activity levels, the presence of acute and chronic diseases, and non-permanent physical conditions (such as pregnancy, breastfeeding, or injury).

These needs can vary on a day-to-day basis; for example, an individual may need different nutrients on a day where he or she is engaging in a strenuous fitness activity versus a day where the individual is sedentary. In order to set appropriate nutrition targets, the dietetic professional will first consider the client's lifestyle and current health status alongside their health goals. For example, consider a twenty-three-year-old female client with 16 percent body fat, no history of chronic mental or physical health conditions, who weight trains four times a week but is struggling to gain lean muscle mass. In this case, the dietetic professional will likely increase the client's total daily calorie consumption by adding more carbohydrates and protein. This will provide the nutrients needed to fuel the client's extra energy expenditure from weight training, and repair and build muscle tissue for the type of mass increase she desires. A twenty-three-year-old female client with 16 percent body fat, no chronic mental or physical health conditions, who is moderately active each day but struggles to feel full after meals may need a different recommendation. In this example, adjusting the client's caloric intake so that the ratio of carbohydrates is lower, with a higher protein and monounsaturated fat intake, will likely help her feel fuller after meals.

In general, energy balance occurs when the individual expends as much energy (calories) as he or she consumes. However, the balanced consumption of macronutrients is as important for optimal mind and body functioning as caloric consumption and expenditure.

Determining Specific Feeding Needs
Feeding needs can change based on age, health status, health and fitness goals, religious and cultural beliefs, and allergies. For example, breastfeeding babies may nurse on demand, whereas bottle-fed

babies may follow a timed feeding schedule. In infants and toddlers, higher dietary fat consumption is necessary to support rapidly developing brain function. Endurance athletes may require higher carbohydrate levels to support training routines that require quick and constant energy sources. Individuals who are allergic to common protein sources, such as dairy or eggs, may need to find alternatives. Individuals with chronic disorders (such as metabolic syndromes) may need to change their feeding habits to maintain or increase their quality of life. Some cultures may not allow meat consumption; therefore, these individuals may need to find different complete protein and B12 sources.

Many secondary health issues may relate back to the individual's nutrition intake. A detailed food diary (which records foods eaten, times eaten, mental response, and physical response) provides data to analyze what nutrients may be missing or are being consumed in excess. This information can help tailor a nutrition plan that meets the client's needs.

Composition/Texture of Foods

Foods are primarily comprised of the main macronutrients: fat, carbohydrates, and protein. Within these, the nutrients are broken down further into fatty acids, fiber, and amino acids. Foods can be consumed in solid, pureed, liquid, or supplement form.

Dietary fat assists with the absorption of some vitamins, contributes to feelings of satiety, and plays a role in healthy skin. In general, a diet high in saturated fat and all trans-fats should be avoided, as these are associated with high cholesterol levels and cardiovascular diseases. Sources of unsaturated fat, such as olive oils, nuts, and fatty fish, are healthier options that consist of omega fatty acids, which support brain health and high-density lipoprotein ("good cholesterol") profiles. Omega fatty acids can also be consumed in supplement form, but this is usually more difficult for the body to absorb and utilize. There are nine calories in one gram of fat.

Dietary carbohydrates are a source of energy, as these macronutrients are easily stored and quickly break down into glucose molecules. They also play an important role in fluid homeostasis. Carbohydrates can be found in most foods, and are most concentrated in starchy and sugary foods. Obtaining carbohydrates from fibrous whole foods such as starchy tubers (like sweet potatoes) and minimally processed grains (such as steel-cut oats) is a healthier option than highly processed sugary foods (such as cakes), which can cause metabolic disorders and contribute to cardiovascular problems. There are four calories in one gram of carbohydrate.

Proteins are crucial macronutrients that are the basis of every cellular structure in the body. Proteins primarily repair and build cells in the body. Upon consumption, they are broken down into chains of amino acids. Healthy sources of proteins are found in animal meat, dairy products, eggs, fish, beans, and nuts. There are four calories in one of gram of protein.

Finally, foods may also include vitamins, minerals, and/or phytonutrients. Vitamins and minerals need water or fat in which to dissolve before they can be utilized. They assist with hundreds of refined human processes such as cellular and skeletal repair, disease protection and prevention, metabolism, and digestion. Phytonutrients are natural plant-based antioxidants and anti-inflammatories that provide different immunity benefits than macronutrients, vitamins, and minerals.

Sources and Preparation Standards

The United States Food and Drug Administration (FDA) is the regulatory authority that oversees the sourcing and preparation of foods sold publicly for consumption in the United States. Its purpose is to ensure that the public receives safe, non-contaminated food for consumption. The FDA establishes and enforces guidelines for what legally constitutes as a food processing and distribution facility, sets guidelines for consumable animal and plant products, determines if and how additives can be utilized in the food, and dictates how foods can be received, stored, and sold publicly by vendors. In addition, the FDA regulates how vendors handle food, the training that should be received by all vendor staff, the ways in which cross-contamination should be contained, and the type and frequency of food-related records that should be kept. Violations of these sourcing and preparation guidelines can result in penalties or facility shutdown.

Modified Diet Products

Personal health statuses or health goals may require some clients to have modified diets; that is, diets that add, reduce, or eliminate specific nutrients. One example of the need for a modified diet is that of an individual who has severe food allergies. Common allergens include nuts, eggs, dairy, gluten, and artificial or synthetic additives. In this instance, the client would need to eliminate the allergenic food and possibly replace it with an alternative nutrient source. In the United States, there are many options for alternative nutrient sources. For example, individuals who are allergic to dairy products can find milks, cheeses, and non-dairy desserts made from soy and nut milks. A wide array of gluten-free products exists; the gluten protein is often replaced with other binders, such as guar gum, xanthan gum, pectin, or binding-type seeds. Many food companies are cognizant of common allergens, and therefore indicate on their packaging whether a food product is free of common food allergens or if the product was processed in a facility where common food allergens are present.

Other situations that would require modified diet products include the presence of cardiovascular or metabolic diseases. In individuals making lifestyle changes to combat cardiovascular diseases, a cholesterol-free diet may be recommended. Individuals with metabolic disorders may need to choose foods low in processed sugar, or utilize low-glycemic sweeteners such as agave or coconut palm sugar.

Enteral Feedings

Enteral feedings refer to tubal feedings, usually administered when an individual is physically unable or otherwise unwilling to feed oneself a nutritionally balanced diet. These types of feedings are commonly seen in severely ill or debilitated patients, pre- or post-operative patients, or malnourished patients. Enteral feedings can vary based on tubal placement and the type of food that is delivered.

Nasoenteric feeding tubes are placed into the nose. Nasogastric feeding tubes are directed from the nasal cavity into the stomach. Nasoduodenal and nasojejunal feeding tubes are directed from the nasal cavity into the small intestine. In some cases, especially when enteral feeding may be necessary for months at a time, a tube may be placed directly into the stomach (percutaneous endoscopic gastrostomy) or small intestine (percutaneous endoscopic jejunostomy).

Formulations for enteral feedings can be commercially prepared (therefore following a standardized nutrient composition). These preparations generally follow a composition of 10 to 15% proteins, 50 to 60% carbohydrates, and 30 to 35% fats. Using these requires that the patient have some digestive ability; for patients that can only perform limited digestive processes, feedings consist of broken down molecules (i.e., amino acids, glucose, and fatty acids). Tailored formulations are utilized when certain diseases are present that require different nutritional intake. For example, in patients with kidney disease, enteral feedings may have different levels of electrolytes in order to ease organ stress. Patients with compromised immune systems or wounds may receive enteral feedings that are higher in immunity-boosting antioxidants (such as glutamine or vitamin C).

Enteral feedings may take place continuously with a drip or pump, or intermittently (known as bolus feeding). Bolus feedings are typically only used with tubes placed directly into the stomach and are primarily recommended for lower-risk patients. When administering enteral feedings, practitioners should be mindful of abdominal bloating, diarrhea, constipation, or other gastrointestinal issues, as these can indicate feeding problems.

Food Supplements

Food supplements are commonly used in the United States. These supplements usually add vitamins, minerals, phytonutrients, amino acids, or herbs to an individual's diet. They can come in pill form, powder form, tea bags, or pre-made shakes. While it is recommended that people try to obtain as many of these as necessary through natural food sources, supplementation can help in areas of deficiency and consequently manage health issues. For example, calcium supplements may be recommended for individuals with osteopenia to mitigate acceleration of the disease. Anemic patients may be prescribed iron supplements. Folic acid supplementation in pregnant women may prevent birth defects. The efficacy of supplements is not regulated by any public agencies. However, the FDA has established Good Manufacturing Practices (GMP) for supplement companies to follow and checks facilities from time to time. U.S. Pharmacopeia, Consumer Lab, and NSF International are three well-known organizations that offer quality testing; the approval of one of these (usually a visible logo on the supplement package) indicates that the supplement is unlikely to cause harm but, again, does not guarantee the efficacy of the product. Dietetic professionals should be prepared to help clients pick reputable supplements that can reliably aid in desired health goals.

Methods of Nourishment

Nourishment occurs in different ways. People can choose to consume raw foods, cooked foods, or a combination of the two. Nutrition can be found in liquid form through drinks such as shakes, juices, and smoothies. People can choose to adopt various diets or styles of eating, such as vegetarian, vegan, plant-based, Mediterranean, Paleo, whole foods, low-carb, high-carb, ketogenic, or standard American. More restrictive styles of eating may produce intended health, fitness, or physical results, but can be harder to maintain long-term. For optimal health, it is recommended that the average healthy person eat a wide variety of whole foods across all macronutrients: lean proteins (such as fish, chicken, turkey, beans, or nuts), fibrous, low-sugar, minimally processed carbohydrates (such as whole grains, vegetables, and fruits), and monounsaturated fats (such as avocados, seed oils, and nut butters).

Routes

The oral route of nutrition is the standard method of food consumption for most average, healthy individuals. Digestion begins by placing food in the mouth, chewing, allowing enzymes in the saliva to break down the food, and using the tongue and jaw to move the food down the throat, through the esophagus, stomach, and intestines. Liquid consumption follows the same route, though chewing is unnecessary.

The enteral route of nutrition refers to any type of food consumption that takes place directly through the path mentioned above, as long as the stomach and intestines are involved in digestive processes. It can also include tubal feeding. The parenteral route involves directing nutrients to the body while bypassing the stomach and intestines, commonly used when the individual suffers from gastrointestinal disease (such as Crohn's or bowel obstruction) that would prevent enteral feeding. Parenteral route is performed intravenously, is costly and time consuming, and requires a medical facility (or a team of medical professionals and equipment, should parenteral feeding occur at home).

Techniques/Equipment

Enteral feeding may require tubes or catheters. In these instances, a surgeon or radiologist and surgical tools are required. Parenteral feeding requires intravenous drip equipment (such as short- or long-term catheters) and qualified medical personnel to administer feedings.

Values/Limitations/Complications

Enteral feeding is a valuable option for pre- and post-operative patients or other contexts where the patient is unable to orally consume food. Enteral feeding has the advantage of using existing digestive abilities to absorb delivered nutrients. Parenteral feeding is a valuable option for those suffering from gastrointestinal diseases or failures, or who voluntarily refuse to eat. There are few limitations to enteral feeding; most people who need to receive nutrients this way are able to; they can even administer nutrients this way at home. Qualified professionals or a team must administer parenteral feeding in a clinical setting, and equipment must be delivered to the outpatient setting. Complications of enteral feeding include irritation or infection at the site of the tube placement, diarrhea, constipation, nausea, and electrolyte/vitamin/mineral imbalances. Complications of parenteral feeding include irritation or infection at the site of the catheter, blood clots, or catheter blockages. Changing the composition of the food, administering electrolyte or other supplementation, and continuous antibiotic treatment while feeding occurs may treat these complications.

Diet Patterns/Schedules and/or Specific Meals for Diagnostic Tests (e.g., Test Meals)

Nutritional diagnostic tests are often used in the case of food allergies and food sensitivities. In these instances, an elimination diet may be used where the client removes one food at a time (usually common allergens or irritants such as gluten, eggs, dairy, sugar, nightshade vegetables) for a pre-determined duration, and records any changes in health or symptom status. Additionally, a reintroduction diet may be utilized, in which a client eliminates ALL potential irritants for a pre-determined duration, and reintroduces suspect foods one at a time to notice if symptoms reoccur. Finally, diet patterns may change for regular health tests, such as lipid panel testing (requires fasting blood work), glucose testing in pregnancy (requires fasting blood work, the ingestion of glucose, and follow-up blood work), or pre-operative fasting (due to the use of anesthesia).

Documentation of Client Care

As in all healthcare fields, documentation of client care should remain confidential and secure. For a nutrition client, a dietetic technician may be responsible for collecting and documenting initial intake information, such as client consent to care, personal demographics, medical history, insurance information, and treatment goals. Other documentation may include appointment frequency and duration, educational counseling that occurred, patient mood assessments, patient assignments, goals for the next session, any ordered tests, blood work results, and/or referrals to other specialists. Documenting these items allows the practitioner to easily compile the client's progress, notice trends, and effectively communicate with other medical providers who serve the client.

PES Statements

A Problems, Etiology, and Symptoms (PES) statement is a goal-oriented mission statement created by a dietitian to clearly communicate the client's reason for seeking treatment. It is usually a brief, one- to two-sentence statement that covers the presenting nutrition related problem, what is causing the problem, and evidence to support the diagnosis. An example PES statement may read as: "High blood glucose levels indicating pre-diabetic conditions relating to over-consumption of high sugar foods and excess body fat percentage, as evidenced by fasting and non-fasting blood glucose levels exceeding 126 mg/dL, client food log, and established medical history."

Other Methodology and Procedures

Another methodology encountered in the dietetic practice may include the Nutrition Care Model, the primary theoretical model utilized in this field. This model focuses on the dynamic between the practitioner and the client, taking into account the training and ethical conduct brought to the relationship by the practitioner, as well as the factors in the client's life and environment that would allow the client to benefit from this working relationship. Within the Nutrition Care Model, dietetic practitioners will likely utilize the **Nutrition Care Process (NCP)**. This systematic framework allows practitioners to understand the client's nutritional history and nutritional goals in a way that will allow them to deliver tailored, targeted interventions. The NCP utilizes an evidence-based approach to provide care. The steps to follow in this framework include a) the nutrition assessment, where medical history as it pertains to nutrition is collected, b) diagnosis, which typically includes a PES statement, c) intervention, selected to address the etiology of the presenting problem, and d) monitoring/evaluation, where the practitioner notices how symptoms are responding to the intervention and how treatment should progress.

Implementing Care Plans
Effective care plans are comprehensive, often consisting of prescribed intervention, clinical and personal support staff for the client, ongoing education, continuity of care, referrals to other modalities of healthy living, and ongoing evaluation.

Provision of Individualized Nutrition Care for Specific Nutrition-Related Problems
The registered dietetic technician helps the practitioner tailor treatment by client and by problem. This framework allows for data collection related to individual history, current nutrition intake, and diet patterns. It highlights areas where there may be nutritional deficiencies or excesses. Additionally, it provides a reliable baseline against which to measure how the intervention is working.

Communication Regarding Plans

Other Healthcare Personnel
These members can play a crucial role in a client's intervention (i.e. a psychologist may be able to help a client address eating behaviors that are leading to a nutrient deficiency); therefore, efficient cross-communication is important. This can be achieved by maintaining detailed documentation of a client's history, sessions, treatments, and goals. Electronic records, rather than paper records, can be helpful when a team of various healthcare personnel is delivering a client's intervention, as these allow real-time updates that everyone can view. Rounding allows different team members to maintain a relationship with the client, and care conferences allow members an established time during which to regularly meet and discuss the client's needs, treatment plan, and prognosis.

Patients and Families, Including Informed Consent
All adult clients will need to provide informed consent to treatment before beginning any interaction or receiving any treatment from healthcare personnel. If the client is incapacitated, under the age of eighteen, or otherwise unable to give consent, an appointed guardian may act on the client's behalf. Additionally, the client must give permission to healthcare personnel to share relevant health information with family members or close friends. Often, these groups act as vital support systems for the client and are involved in the treatment process, but the client must be comfortable with these support systems having the knowledge of his or her medical history. This protects the client's rights to privacy and dignity.

Educate
In order to best educate clients, the practitioner should develop the care plan around the client's needs and goals. Additionally, the practitioner should empower the client to be an active participant in their nutrition goals. Providing in-depth nutrition education not only to the client, but also to the client's support system can better help the client reach his or her goals. Finally, the practitioner should emphasize how nutrition changes can and should be viewed as an active and ongoing lifestyle

modification for positive change, rather than a "restrictive diet" which can feel more negative for the client.

Discharge Planning for Continuity of Care

Discharge planning, in these instances, is often a comprehensive team effort. As discharge paperwork is prepared, the practitioner should notate the role of nutrition in the client's future plans and goals. This may include a detailed nutrition plan, the objectives and goals of the plan, and the practical applications that the client needs to embrace in order to sustain their habits and work toward goals. It is good practice to verbally review this paperwork with the client before discharge and provide contact information for any follow-up questions that arise.

Recommend Clients Receive Physical, Social, Behavioral and Psychological Services

Healthy nutrition is a component of overall wellness. Good nutrition correlates with physical benefits (such as healthy body weight), social benefits (such as when parents cook healthy meals at home and eat with their children, correlated with healthier and happier families), and behavioral and psychological benefits (such as calm behaviors and stable moods). Comparatively, when clients receive medical guidance to improve nutrition intake and habits, addressing their physical, social, behavioral, and psychological health and habits is also an important component of reaching and sustaining health goals. These aspects of life can hinder or support reaching nutrition goals. For example, poor physical health may affect nutrition absorption. Poor social support may prove to be an obstacle for making diet changes. Poor behavioral and psychological habits may trigger previous detrimental eating habits.

Documenting Implementation

Documentation practices may vary by location, so thoroughly familiarizing oneself with the standard operating procedures of the facility where one works is crucial. For example, some facilities may document all client information electronically, while others still utilize paper-charting methods. Typically, documenting includes details records of client medical history, appointments, cancellations, creating reports, evaluating data, and analyzing how well treatment is working. Maintaining detailed records also helps dietetic technicians communicate better with the dietitian, maintain accountability, and illustrate technician competency. All client information is considered confidential. Records should be accessible to the client if requested, barring an ethical implication (such as a client who has the potential to do harm to oneself or another with the information).

Interventions for Populations

Specific Diet Types

Therapeutic

A therapeutic diet is one that is prescribed by a physician specifically for the individual patient. This type of diet will be different for each patient, depending on their needs. Normally, a patient on a therapeutic diet will be staying in a facility where specific menu items are served, so the menu will need to be changed and adapted according to the prescribed diet. There are many medical professionals that can contribute to the development of a therapeutic diet for the patient, but only a physician can prescribe this type of diet. A diet manual can also assist the physician in preparing his or her dietary orders. The dietitian or dietary manager must then follow this order and oversee the proper implementations of the prescription. Any changes, modifications, or cancellations of the diet order must come from the doctor, and any questions regarding the diet must be directed to them as well.

High Calorie, High Protein
A high calorie, high protein diet will most often be prescribed for individuals who have lost a significant amount of weight in a short amount of time or those who have been on an enteral or parenteral feeding system for an extended period of time. This type of diet may also be ordered for infants with failure to thrive. In most cases, cancer patients will be ordered to follow a high calorie, high protein diet so that they are better able to maintain their strength and avoid extreme fatigue throughout their treatment. This diet usually includes foods such as whole-fat dairy products (ice cream, milk, butter, yogurt, and cream), peanut butter, meats, nuts, eggs, avocado, and other similar types of foods.

Lactose Intolerance
Lactose intolerance is the inability to break down lactose, the primary sugar found in milk products. For an individual with lactose intolerance, it is important to avoid dairy products that cause symptoms such as upset stomach, diarrhea, bloating, and cramps, but avoidance of dairy products may put the individual at risk of inadequate calcium intake, so this nutrient should be consumed from other sources such as broccoli, dark leafy greens, soy, tofu, salmon, sardines, beans, oranges, and calcium-fortified breads and juices. Certain yogurts contain bacteria cultures that are needed to breakdown lactose, so some individuals may be able to tolerate this. It should be noted that lactose can also be found in nondairy items such as processed foods, vitamins, supplements, and prescription drugs, so it is important for individuals suffering from this intolerance to be aware of this possibility in order to avoid symptoms. Nondairy substitutes such as soy, rice, almond milks, or yogurt products are also available for lactose intolerant individuals.

Vegetarian
Vegetarian diets are plant-based diets that are typically followed by an individual voluntarily. An individual following a vegetarian diet may fall into one of three categories: a *vegan* diet excludes all animal meats and products, including eggs, dairy, and honey; a *lacto-vegetarian* diet allows for the consumption of dairy products; and a *lacto-ovo-vegetarian* diet allows for the consumption of dairy and eggs. It is important for any type of vegetarian to ensure they are receiving an adequate amount of calcium, protein, iron, and vitamin B-12. Foods such as tofu, soy, nuts, nut butters, and enriched cereal and other grain products are helpful in reaching protein and calcium requirements for a vegetarian.

Low Cholesterol
A low cholesterol diet is typically followed in order to reduce the risk of cardiovascular disease, by controlling and reducing levels of cholesterol and blood lipids. The target daily intake of an individual following a low cholesterol diet is about 200 to 300 milligrams of cholesterol per day. There are two types of cholesterol, which is described as a waxy substance found in the cells. High-density lipoproteins (HDL), or "good" cholesterol, transports cholesterol into the liver, where it is processed and removed from the body. Low density lipoproteins (LDL), or "bad" cholesterol, can lead to a buildup of the waxy substance in arterial walls, forming plaques, which harden the arteries and reduce the diameter available for blood flow. It is important to have a healthy balance of both types of cholesterol, but the body actually synthesizes sufficient cholesterol to meet its needs. Food sources of cholesterol include animal products such as meat, poultry, eggs, seafood, and dairy products. Cholesterol is not found in plant products. A patient following a low cholesterol diet will need to eliminate or drastically reduce the amount of animal products consumed and choose only very lean meat and low fat dairy products. Adding more fruits, vegetables, and whole grains to the diet will also help the individual reduce dietary cholesterol.

Kosher

A Kosher diet is followed by those of the Orthodox Jewish religion and must comply with rules derived from the ancient biblical texts. Within these texts, some foods are permitted while some are not. For example, meats must meet strict requirements regarding the types of animals they come from. A rabbi must oversee the slaughtering of the animal, and it must be done in a humane and painless manner. Meats that are approved in a kosher diet include cow, lamb, chicken, veal, turkey, goat, and duck while pork, shellfish, shrimp, catfish, and any type of insect are not permitted. Kosher regulations also state that any type of dairy cannot come into contact with meat products. There are also rules involving cheese, wine, eggs, fruits, and vegetables. Nutrition professionals should recognize these rules for a patient following a kosher diet and should look for foods labeled as kosher. A single non-kosher ingredient or source can make the entire product or recipe non-kosher.

Islamic

Those practicing a Muslim religion also follow a strict dietary system known as Halal. The Halal diet is similar to the Kosher diet. Pork products, carnivorous and omnivorous animals, certain fowl, non-amphibious animals, blood products, and alcohol are forbidden in the Halal diet. Similar to the Kosher diet, all slaughtering of animals must be humane, painless, and overseen by an expert. Again, a nutrition professional must be aware of these restrictions when working with an Islamic patient and must take care not to include non-Halal ingredients or sources in their diet.

Ketogenic Diet

A ketogenic diet is often used to treat epilepsy or seizure disorders. The high fat content of the diet leads to the fats being converted into ketones that are used as an energy source in place of glucose. Carbohydrates are decreased with this type of diet, resulting in lack of glucose available as an energy source. This leads to improved insulin resistance and an elevated level of ketones, or ketosis, which can help to reduce episodes of epileptic seizures. It is important to closely monitor the consumption of carbohydrates in the diet, due to the fact that even a small change in sugar levels can disrupt glucose and ketone levels in the body. For most patients following this diet, folate, B6, B12, vitamin D, and calcium supplementation will be necessary.

Hemodialysis Diet

A hemodialysis diet is designed for patients who are in stage 5 of chronic kidney disease (CKD), also referred to as end stage renal disease (ESRD). Patients at this stage of kidney disease have little to no remaining kidney function, so they require dialysis to remove excess waste and fluid from the blood. Hemodialysis, a particular type of dialysis, is usually performed a few times a week for about three to four hours at a time. It requires a specific diet plan meant to decrease the amount of fluid and waste that may build up between hemodialysis treatments. Foods containing high amounts of sodium, phosphorus, and potassium are restricted, and protein intake is increased to a recommended 1.2 g/ kg per day on the diet.

Peritoneal Dialysis Diet

Peritoneal dialysis (PD) is an alternate form of dialysis, which requires a slightly different diet from the hemodialysis diet, to account for differences in the treatments. For example, peritoneal dialysis is performed daily, so there is less buildup of fluid and waste, allowing for a diet with fewer restrictions, particularly regarding sodium and fluid intake. Because protein is lost through the peritoneal membrane and patients are at risk of infections, increased protein intake is needed to keep the patient strong. Recommended protein intake for patients following this diet is 1.2 to 1.3 g protein per kilogram of body weight per day. Peritoneal dialysis patients may experience low potassium levels, so potassium-rich foods such as tomatoes, bananas, and orange juice are encouraged.

Metabolic Disorders
Galactosemia describes two different metabolic syndromes that cause the body to be unable to convert galactose to glucose due to a genetic mutation that affects the galactose-1-phosphate uridyl transferase enzyme, which is needed to break down galactose. Galactose is a simple sugar found in many foods such as celery, beets, and cherries. Type 1, or classic galactosemia, is the most common and most severe form of the condition. If not diagnosed at birth, infants may experience failure to thrive, feeding difficulties, jaundice, lack of energy, sepsis, susceptibility to infections, and nausea. Type 2, or galactokinase deficiency, causes fewer and less severe medical problems. Nutritional intervention for this condition requires elimination of foods containing galactose, including dairy products, dates, bell peppers, organ meats, and papaya.

Urea cycle defects, such as OTC deficiency, citrullinemia, and Argininosuccinic aciduria can cause ammonia to accumulate in the blood, leading to nausea, seizures, or death. Nutritional management may include elimination of all protein from the diet.

Long-Term Care
After the patient is admitted to a long-term care facility, an initial assessment must be completed within the first two weeks. Within a week following the assessment, a care plan, including dietary orders such as special therapeutic diets, is developed for the patient. Therefore, within three weeks of admittance into long-term care, the patient should have a personalized plan of care. This plan should be updated at least quarterly, or as any changes occur.

Cholesterol Management
The National Cholesterol Education Program's clinical guidelines for cholesterol management are periodically updated and presented in the Adult Treatment Panel III (ATP). These reports are compiled from evidence-based research analyzing cholesterol testing and prevention on coronary heart disease.

Currently, a high level of LDL cholesterol continues to be the main factor thought to contribute to heart disease. In order to determine the risk of heart disease, a complete lipoprotein profile should be completed for adults over the age of twenty, and LDL levels should ideally be less than 100 mg/dL. Individuals with risk factors such as smoking, hypertension, diabetes, and family history of CHD should follow a diet low in saturated fat (less than 7 percent of calories) and cholesterol (less than 200 mg/day) and high in fiber (10 to 25 g/day). These individuals should also aim for thirty minutes of moderate intensity exercise on at least five days per week and maintenance of a healthy body weight.

ADA Nutrition Care Process
A medical doctor for patients at risk of nutrition-related issues usually initiates the Nutrition Care Process (NCP). The process includes assessment of nutritional status, diagnosis of nutritional needs, implementation of interventions developed to address nutritional care needs, and monitoring and evaluation of nutritional care. The reason for developing a nutrition care process is to give dietitians a common structure to develop a plan and to validate the care they provide.

Dietary Guides and Their Use
DRI/RDA
Dietary Reference Intake (DRI) is a broad term that guides how an individual plans his or her nutritional intake. DRI varies based on biological and lifestyle factors, as well as health goals. It includes different reference values, such as Adequate Intake (AI), Tolerable Upper Limits (UA), and Acceptable Macronutrient Distribution Ranges (AMDR). Recommended Dietary Allowance (RDA) is a more commonly seen component of one's DRI. It provides a general recommendation of nutrients to consume

to satisfy the average person's needs. Most nutrition labels provide Daily Value guidelines for a 2000-calorie diet; this measure is very similar to the RDA and shows what percentage of daily nutrient that particular food provides.

Again, these amounts may vary by individual. For example, the RDA for calcium for a toddler is approximately 700 mg, while it is 1300 mg for teenagers, and 1000 for young adults. The RDA for Vitamin D stays the same throughout life (600 mg) until older adulthood, where the recommendation increases to 800 mg.

DRI and RDA guidelines are established by the U.S. National Academy of Sciences, through the Institute of Medicine.

Food Group Plans

Meal Planning Applications

There are a number of health-related applications that can be used for meal planning including the United States Department of Agriculture (USDA) Food Patterns, the DASH (Dietary Approaches to Stop Hypertension) Eating Plan, MyPlate, food exchanges, and the glycemic index.

USDA Food Patterns

There are three USDA Food Patterns included in the 2015 – 2020 Dietary Guidelines: Healthy U.S. Style Eating, Healthy Mediterranean Style Eating, and Healthy Vegetarian Style Eating. One eating pattern is not necessarily superior to another, but rather more of a preference; however, a vegetarian lifestyle has been associated with a decreased risk for some chronic diseases such as heart disease and certain cancers. The USDA Food Patterns are based on systematic review from scientific research, food pattern modeling, and analysis of intake of the U.S. population. Each USDA Food Pattern is based on the five food groups—vegetables, fruits, grains, dairy, and protein—and can be customized to meet an individual's needs based on age, sex, height, weight, and level of physical activity.

The Healthy U.S. Style Eating Pattern is based on typical foods consumed in Americans' diets with a focus on nutrient-dense foods in portions that are appropriate for the desired caloric intake. The Healthy Mediterranean Style Eating Pattern is based on the Healthy U.S. Style Eating Pattern but adjusted to align with the eating patterns of the Mediterranean diet, which have been associated with positive health outcomes. Specifically, the Healthy Mediterranean Style Eating Pattern has more fruit and seafood but less dairy than the U.S. Style Eating Pattern. The Healthy Vegetarian Style Eating Pattern is also based on the Healthy U.S. Style Eating Pattern but is adjusted to reflect the eating habits of self-reported vegetarians, as identified in the National Health and Nutrition Examination Survey (NHANES).

Dash Eating Plan for hypertension + lowering LDL

The DASH Eating Plan is based on clinical research trials, which found that the plan helped individuals lower their blood pressure and low-density lipoprotein (LDL) cholesterol and improve heart health, while meeting nutrient requirements. The DASH Eating Plan emphasizes whole grains, poultry, fish, and nuts along with food sources of potassium, calcium, and magnesium. Individuals are encouraged to consume as much as seven to eight servings of grains and four to five servings of fruits and vegetables per day on a 2000-calorie diet. Individuals using the DASH Eating Plan may need to gradually increase the intake of whole grains, fruits, and vegetables, since the increased fiber of these foods can lead to bloating and diarrhea.

MyPlate

The United States Department of Agriculture (USDA) recently developed MyPlate to replace the previous Food Pyramid, a recommendation that the USDA had utilized from 1992 to 2013. This visual intends to help people easily eyeball their portions on a plate, rather than tediously measure out portions. MyPlate recommends a percentage breakdown of 30/40/10/20 corresponding to grains, vegetables, fruits, and lean protein. It also includes a small circle to represent dairy. Variations of this plan exist where dairy is excluded, protein portions are smaller, and monounsaturated fats are included. Essentially, MyPlate is a tool developed by the USDA based on the five food groups and healthy eating, focused on variety, appropriate portion sizes, nutrient-dense foods, and low saturated fat, sodium, and added sugar intake. The MyPlate Daily Checklist and the SuperTracker are two specific online tools that allow individuals to customize nutrition planning for their specific needs.

Food Exchanges

Food exchanges are used for meal planning purposes, especially for those with diabetes and/or seeking weight loss. Food exchanges divide food into six categories based on the amount of carbohydrate, fat, and protein they contain: starches/breads, fruits, milk, vegetables, meat, and fat.

- Starches and breads contain 15 grams of carbohydrate and 3 grams of protein per exchange with 80 calories.

- Fruits contain 15 grams of carbohydrate per exchange with 60 calories.

- Milk exchanges contain 12 grams of carbohydrate; 8 grams of protein; 3 to 8 grams of fat depending on whether the milk exchange is a low-, medium-, or high-fat choice; and 90 to 150 calories depending on the fat content.

- Vegetable exchanges contain 5 grams of carbohydrate per serving with 25 calories.

- Meat exchanges contain 7 grams of protein per ounce and 0 to 8 grams of fat, depending on whether the source of the meat exchange is very lean, lean, medium fat, or high fat with a range of 35 to 100 calories.

- Fat exchanges provide 5 grams of fat and 45 calories.

Glycemic Index

Finally, the glycemic index and glycemic load offer insight as to how foods affect blood glucose and insulin levels. Glycemic index and load can be useful tools in meal planning to help individuals better understand the impact specific foods may have on their blood sugar. Carbohydrate counting may also be a useful tool in helping individuals monitor and understand the impact various carbohydrates have on their blood sugar.

Meal Planning Approaches

Each of these meal-planning approaches are useful in working with clients to guide them toward healthy eating. The most appropriate meal planning approach depends on the client's nutrition goals and personal preferences. For example, a client wanting to lower blood pressure and blood lipids may be best served with the DASH approach. Another individual who would like to adopt a vegetarian lifestyle may be more interested in using the USDA Healthy Vegetarian Style Eating Pattern, while a client hoping to lower blood sugar might be interested in food exchanges and/or the glycemic index as a meal planning approach.

Federal Dietary Guidelines and Goals

The USDA and the United States Department of Health and Human Services (HHS) publishes specific reports to help guide healthy dietary choices in the population.

Dietary Guidelines for Americans

This report is published every five years to provide healthcare and public health clinicians, educators, researchers, and policy makers with the most recent nutrition science updates, research, and recommendations in order to help them develop media and materials that will assist the population in making educated food and diet decisions. The current edition (8th) is valid from 2015 to 2020. The goal of this document is for health promotion, chronic disease prevention, and healthy weight maintenance as it pertains to nutritional intake. This version is the first to incorporate how behavior, such as eating patterns, influence nutritional choices. Current and prior *Dietary Guidelines* can be downloaded for free in PDF format at www.health.gov.

Surgeon General's Report on Nutrition and Health

The first *Surgeon General's Report on Nutrition and Health* was published in 1988 as a 700-page document that outlines research related to nutrition and chronic disease. This report stated that the population should limit fat, sugar, and sodium in order to prevent obesity and disease. However, obesity rates and chronic disease rates continue to rise. This trend was an important influencer in pushing the USDA and HHS to tailor nutritional recommendations by creating MyPlate, which helped with portion control and other healthful eating habits. In addition, some new dietary recommendations shift some of the chronic disease blame to sugar-laden, highly processed carbohydrates and suggest that moderate doses of healthy fats are crucial in a balanced diet. Overall, new reports emphasize the portion and quality of a food (i.e., organic, minimally processed), rather than considering calories and single nutrients, for better health.

National Groups

Most recognized national health groups emphasize the importance of nutrient-dense diets paired with moderate to high physical activity levels. Each of the organizations below also provides printable handouts of meal plans and portion size examples on their websites.

National Heart, Lung & Blood Institute (NHLBI)

The NHLBI, a unit of the National Institutes of Health (a division of the HHS), focuses on health promotion and diseases relating to the heart, lungs, and blood. The NHLBI is a proponent of the Dietary Approaches to Stop Hypertension (DASH) eating plan, which is a flexible eating plan that supports heart health. In general, the DASH eating plans advocates for the consumption of primarily vegetables, fruits, and whole grains while limiting sugars, sodium, and sources of saturated fats such as meat, dairy, and oils. The DASH diet also focuses on incorporating high amounts of potassium, calcium, fiber, and lean protein. This way of eating has been associated with lower risk and/or decreased progression of heart disease, kidney stones, kidney disease, and diabetes.

American Cancer Society

The American Cancer Society (ACS) is committed to the research and education of cancer treatment, management, and prevention. The organization publishes dietary guidelines that may help prevent or manage cancers. This includes maintaining low body fat, limiting sugar and alcohol, and making nutritional choices focusing on whole and plant foods. Additionally, the ACS recommends eating organic foods when possible and limiting the use of synthetic preservatives and additives in foods.

American Heart Association (AHA)

The AHA focuses on the research and education regarding cardiovascular health. The organization recommends including fruits, vegetables, whole grains, beans, legumes, nuts, seeds, lean meats or plant proteins, healthy fats and oils, and minimal dairy. AHA recommends limiting sodium, saturated and trans fat, sugar, and red meat.

National Cholesterol Education Program

This program is managed by NHLBI and focuses specifically on lowering cholesterol levels with the end goal of lowering cardiovascular disease rates. This program recommends testing cholesterol levels regularly and following the Therapeutic Lifestyles Change (TLC) diet. This diet emphasizes limiting red meat, dairy products, and generally choosing a plant-based diet.

Breastfeeding initiatives

A number of organizations, such as the American Academy of Pediatrics (AAP), the World Health Organization (WHO), and La Leche League (LLL) promote breastfeeding initiatives to educate and support mothers and families in breastfeeding infants. For the child, exclusive breastfeeding for the first six months of life and breastfeeding paired with healthy solids from six months to toddlerhood support the child's immune system, development of hunger and satiety cues, emotional needs, and palate refinement. Breastfeeding also encourages oxytocin release in the mother (associated with maternal relaxation, positive mood, and mother-baby bonding) and may lower the mother's risk of breast cancer. Exclusively breastfeeding mothers need to eat nutrient-dense, balanced diets and consume approximately 500 extra calories per day in order to produce ample, high-quality milk.

Other

Other groups that focus on population nutrition include:

- The Academy of Nutrition and Dietetic, which provide dietary advice for many demographics (i.e., pregnant women, immunosuppressed populations, those with food allergies, etc.) based on the most current research

- The National Alliance for Nutrition and Activity, which supports laws and interest groups focused on improving population health through healthy eating and exercise

- The American Nutrition Association, which promotes wellness through nutrition education

Within communities, hospitals, clinics, and pharmacies also regularly provide nutrition guidance and counseling services.

Community Nutrition Programs Services and Implementation

Public assistance programs provide food and nutrition services to at-risk populations. These programs are often funded by federal, state, private, and/or non-profit dollars. They can provide benefits such as subsidized groceries, meal delivery, or nutrition education.

Federal Resources and Food Assistance Programs

SNAP (Supplemental Nutrition Assistance Program)

The Food Stamp Program provide low income individuals with coupons and debit cards to be used to purchase healthy foods. Reimbursements are provided based on foods that meet dietary guidelines at a low cost. To be eligible to participate, individuals and families must prove that they fall below the poverty line as well as the minimum amount of countable assets. Breads, cereal, produce, meat, dairy, seeds, or plants that will produce fruits and vegetables are among the items that can be purchased using a food stamp program, but non-food items and hot foods cannot be purchased.

Title III Nutrition Services

This program housed under the Administration of Aging ad provides nutrition services for the elderly. It primarily focuses on individuals over the age of sixty who are low-income, minority, or in other need of social or economic assistance. The mission of the program is to feed and provide socialization for older individuals that may be experiencing food insecurity, poverty, or isolation, and to consequently improve this demographics' health outcome. In addition to utilizing federal resources, many of these programs also have state, local, charitable, and private non-profit support. Overall, it is estimated these initiatives provide close to one million meals daily.

Child Nutrition Programs

Healthy Start and Head Start

The goal of the Healthy Start program is to improve the health of pregnant women and reduce the rate of infant mortality by providing free prenatal care in clinics. Women in between pregnancies can also benefit from counseling or treatment of issues that can complicate future pregnancies, such as obesity, diabetes, or substance abuse.

The Head Start program prepares preschool aged children for school by providing nutritional, social, health, and educational services. Nutrition professionals can contribute to this program by presenting educational programs to the children and teaching parents how to prepare healthy food for their families.

National School Lunch Program

The National School Lunch Program was established by president Truman in 1946 in order to provide free and reduced-cost lunches to qualifying children throughout the nation within public schools, nonprofit private schools, and childcare facilities. Federal subsidies are provided to qualifying schools, provided they serve healthy, well-balanced meals to the students. Children must meet requirements in order to qualify for free or reduced lunches. Children from families with incomes between 130 percent to 185 percent of the poverty level will receive free or reduced cost meals. In addition to government subsidies, schools may receive additional support in the form of commodity foods from the USDA.

The School Breakfast Program, Special Milk Program, and Summer Food Program

The USDA's Food and Nutrition Service serves to provide reimbursements to schools that serve free or reduced cost breakfasts to qualifying students. USDA's Team Nutrition also assists food service staff with menu planning, training, and education.

The Special Milk Program ensures that children who do not participate in any other meal program are still provided with milk. This program encourages the consumption of milk in schools and provides reimbursements for the milk they provide.

The Summer Food Program helps provide up to three meals per day to children during school breaks using sites such as camps and community centers.

Child and Adult Care Food Program (CACFP)

The CACFP provides food to low-income children and disabled elderly individuals who are enrolled in a public or private daycare service or after school program. Individuals in daycare settings can receive up to two meals and one snack per day and those in after school programs can receive one snack per day. Homeless shelters can provide three meals per day to children. Reimbursements can be calculated as a percentage, per meal count, or blended per meal rates. Recipes and purchased commodities are provided by the USDA.

Special Supplemental Nutrition Program for Women, Infants, and Children

WIC Program

The Special Supplemental Nutrition Program for Women, Infants, and Children (WIC) enables qualifying individuals to receive nutritious foods, counseling, education, and referrals to other similar social service programs. Eligibility to participate in the program is determined by the individual's income and level of nutritional risk and pregnant women, women 6-12 months postpartum, and children up to the age of five can participate in the program. Anemia, weight problems, and history of pregnancy complications are indications of nutritional risks. Participants can receive items such as cow's milk, 100% juice, infant formula, and iron-fortified cereal.

Expanded Food and Nutrition Education Program (EFNEP)

The EFNEP is federally funded through the Cooperative Extension Service in each state and US territory. This program provides services to teach families about healthy eating habits, how to save money and still purchase healthy foods, and food safety techniques to reduce the risk of foodborne illness.

Food Banks and Other Community Resources

Commodity Food Donation/Distribution Program

The USDA's Commodity Food Program serves to provide food to individuals in need, as well as to help provide a market for goods produced by American farmers. Nutrition is provided to the populations deemed to be at the highest risk of poor nutrition: low-income women, children under age six, and the elderly. The Commodity Supplemental Food Program can provide items such as canned meats and vegetables, cereal, and juice, but is not meant to provide all nutritional needs.

The Emergency Food Assistance Program provides foods from the USDA to each state to distribute to local food banks, where it is moved to soup kitchens or directly to households for temporary, emergency solution.

SOP, SOPP, and SODPF

The Standards of Practice in Nutrition Care (SOP), Standards of Professional Performance (SOPP), and the Scope of Dietetic Practice Framework (SODPF) all work to support quality dietetic practices according to the philosophy set forth by the Nutrition Care Process and Model. The SOP includes various services and treatments that a nutrition professional can provide safely. The SOPP provides information on satisfactory behavior that a dietitian should exhibit when working in a professional setting. The SODPF is an outline of the knowledge base, ethics, research, education, and standards of care that encompass the dietetic profession. These systems can be used by the nutrition professional to evaluate their own performance, by administration to assure the patient's needs are met, by human resources during the hiring process, and by supervisors to monitor employee's performance.

Healthy People 2020 Program

The Healthy People 2020 program is a collection of goals and objectives from the Surgeon General to encourage the general population to lead healthy lifestyles in order to prevent disease. The information can be used by local governments to develop health-oriented programs within the community. The two main goals of the program are to improve quality of life and to eliminate health disparities. There are twenty-eight areas of focus in this program, ranging from food safety to chronic diseases. The program includes progress markers and objective measurements so that goals can be assessed. An example of a goal included in the Healthy People 2020 program is that children participate in 60 minutes of vigorous physical activity daily in order to prevent obesity.

Lead Education or Support Groups for Client Populations
Registered dietetic technicians play an instrumental role in healthcare delivery by leading education or support groups for their clients, especially for those that have low risk factors. By providing these services, dietetic technicians help the registered focus more on high-risk patients without neglecting the concerns or interests of lower risk clients. This cooperative approach can provide higher quality services to a broader range of patients.

In order to effectively lead education or support groups, it is important for the dietetic technician to be aware of any needs assessments that have been performed by their practice, a framework which indicates which topics the clients are most interested in learning about or are crucial educational topics for their health goals. When the support group has been established and begun meeting, it is important for the leader to set the tone for the group to keep meetings productive, focused, and solution-oriented. It is also important for the leader to be welcoming, positive, open-minded, and a good listener to encourage repeat participation, which in turn will likely help participants achieve their health goals. Finally, it is acceptable to be available to participants between sessions (such as by phone, in-person meetings, or email), but it is vital that the educator places and enforces limits to off-session interactions (such as placing strict off-session hours for these kinds of communication). This encourages participant engagement in the sessions that have been established especially for them, and discourages participants from contacting healthcare providers nonstop.

Distributing Nutrition Information Through the Media
Distributing nutrition information through the media includes sending informational mailers, building websites, running a public service announcement on radio or television, utilizing social media, or giving handouts at educational sessions. Topics covered can include educational information about nutrient consumption (i.e., which foods provide which nutrients, how different nutrients are beneficial or detrimental to the mind and body, eating mindfully) or about food-related programs (i.e., public assistance programs, weight loss programs, healthy eating programs). Topics can also include information about food sourcing, diet trends, and facts and myths about popular diets.

Since this avenue of health communication often caters to wide audiences with varying nutritional needs, it is important that practitioners keep this type of information applicable, reliable, factual, and useful for the audience.

Education and Training

Targeted Audiences
Education and training will vary based on the target audience, so it is important to keep the audience's needs and goals in mind when preparing educational material. Educating a patient may include dietary guidelines and behavior modifications specific to their health goals; the patient may not be there voluntarily, so empowering the patient and gaining the patient's trust will be a key component of the session. A client may be attending sessions voluntarily with a specific goal in mind, and may desire certain information and guidance. Employees may need continuing and ongoing education and training to ensure that they not only know their industry skills, but also are aware of practice policies and operating procedures. Students may want hands-on and applicable education and training that can be utilized in their careers.

Goals and Objectives

When developing goals and objectives for an educational or training session, it is important for the practitioner to note what is medically necessary to achieve, and also what additional outcomes (if any) are desired by the client. Goals should be long-term, accessible achievements. Objectives should be specific, measurable, attainable, and realistic; they should also state a time frame in which they should be met. Multiple detailed objectives should, if achieved, create the pathway to the desired goal.

Education Venue

Education and training can occur in a variety of contexts and settings. They can occur in traditional classroom settings (such as in worksite wellness lunch-and-learn hours), during individual client sessions, through online modalities such as virtual learning modules, informational blogs, and social media, or over the phone with a healthcare provider. Thanks to the advent of technology, the venues in which health and wellness guidance is offered has changed.

Content Specifications

Content should be tailored to the audience that is receiving education and training. For example, a demographic that is less comfortable using technology may be more likely to utilize paper resources (such as a bound food diary), while a demographic that prefers technology may prefer to utilize an online app (such as MyFitnessPal). Both groups, however, may enjoy community events and resources that provide them with the education they are looking for (such as a nutrition counseling booth at the local farmer's market). In general, educational and training content should be enjoyable, accessible, and easy to use for the target audience.

Evaluation Criteria

With any program, it is important to regularly evaluate its components to ensure that the desired outcomes are being achieved and to note how any processes can be improved. Any form of program evaluation should be systematic and clearly illustrate how components of the program influence established outcomes. This analysis may include the need that existed for the program, baseline data, the program's effects (what outcomes indicate that the program is working as intended), what participation in the program entails, what resources are needed, the relationship between resources used and program effects, and how data from the program will be used in the future. In general, concrete data (regardless of whether data is quantitative or qualitative with established parameters) should be utilized.

Budget Development

Budgets should take into account all costs—financial, human, time, materials, etc.—needed to run the program. Many non-profit nutrition programs rely on funding from outside sources, such as federal or charitable grant funds. These applications will require a detailed proposed budget and may award funds based on the proposal's accuracy and evidence of need. Typically, developing the budget should account for the following components:

- Facility and equipment
- Necessary hardware and software
- Facility furnishings and décor
- Security systems (for the building, as well as for client information)
- Personnel salary and benefits for hours worked
- Employee trainings and development opportunities
- Daily, monthly, and annual operating costs (payroll services, facility maintenance, electricity, water, Internet, telephone)

- Cleaning costs
- Material costs (paper, printing)
- Miscellaneous costs if desired (extras such as magazines for the waiting room, water cooler, toys for children)

These should be compared against the expected revenue from services. Costs should be divided into those that are necessary for operations, and those that may be beneficial but are not vital.

Program Promotion

Appropriately and adequately marketing a program is necessary for its success. Effectively promoting a program usually incorporates the 4 P's of marketing: product, price, placement, and promotion. Clients need to know what exactly the program (product) entails, what services are available, and how the program will be of benefit. The cost (price) for the client may be more than financial when it comes to "buying" a health service; it may also include the client's time, travel, and personal development. This trade-off will influence whether or not the client pursues the program. Program accessibility and target audience (placement) is also crucial. If the wrong audience is targeted (i.e., a low risk population for a DASH diet program), future participation is likely to be low. If the program is inaccessible for those who need it (i.e., a high-risk population that is interested in learning more about certain diets, but the program occurs during the holidays), participation is also likely to be low. Programs should be interesting and convenient to use for a targeted audience. Finally, knowing how to cull and reach the targeted audience is an important component of the fourth P (promotion). Programs should be inviting and appropriate for the target audience, and their presence and benefits should be communicated appropriately. For example, a program that takes place through a worksite may be promoted through the company's Intranet, while a town's local program may be promoted through a community center's information board.

Monitoring and Evaluation

National Council Against Health Fraud

The National Council Against Health Fraud is a private and voluntary agency that advocates against misinformation and believes that nutrition products and services should be safe and effective. They fight for consumer health laws, investigate health claims, and educate the public on fraud.

Federal Trade Commission

The Federal Trade Commission (FTC) is a government agency that protects consumers against false health claims and ineffective products. Consumers can file claims with the FTC and request free information concerning health claims.

Monitoring Progress and Updating Previous Care for Uncomplicated Conditions

Monitoring Responses to Nutrition Care

Nutrition monitoring is the continual process of observing a patient to determine the success of a nutrition care plan. Monitoring is crucial to assess whether the patient's status is improving or if it is necessary to update the care plan and take corrective action. Data should be collected and evaluated beginning at the time of implementation and continue regularly for the duration of treatment.

Comparing Outcomes to Nutrition Interventions

Prior to beginning an intervention, the practitioner may establish key indicators that show if the client is on track toward a desired health outcome. These indicators may be divided into food and nutrition knowledge and behavior outcomes (such as knowing and utilizing portion sizes), anthropometric measurement outcomes (such as inches lost), biochemical outcomes (such as lowered triglyceride levels), or physical outcomes (such as increased energy levels). Outcomes may be flexible and can be changed during treatment. For example, a client who seeks treatment wanting to lose a set number of pounds may later be satisfied by lipid panel numbers that fall within a healthy range.

An organization may develop protocols to assist nutritional professionals in the care process. These protocols can be included in the policy and procedures manual to assure that each professional follows the same principles of care and service. This can include step-by-step instructions, treatment timelines, monitoring procedures, lab work, and consultations. Data is gathered from outcome management systems to monitor the efficacy of a treatment plan, while statistical samplings help evaluate treatment procedures for large groups of patients.

Monitoring Medication and Dietary Supplement Use

Medication and dietary supplements are an important component of intervention. They may be prescribed to assist in reaching nutritional goals (such as supplementing vitamins to address a deficiency). Or, they may be acknowledged as having an unintended effect on nutritional goals (such as hormone medications that can suppress appetite). The practitioner should be aware of how medications and dietary supplements can help or hinder a client's progress and incorporate this into the treatment plan.

Monitoring Tolerance of Diet, Tube Feeding and Medical Nutrition Supplements

In this context, practitioners must be mindful of the situation that led the client to needing diet modifications. If a diet modification includes removing or adding foods due to an allergy or intolerance, the practitioner should note any changes that occur with removing or adding each food; the client also plays an important role in adhering to, documenting, and sharing the effects of the modification so that an accurate medical assessment can be made. This is also true when a client begins a new supplement routine. In the instance of tube feeding, side effects such as diarrhea, constipation, pain at the site of the tube, and weight loss are common. Practitioners will need to offer plenty of support by way of modifying the composition of the food in the tube, changing feeding from enteral to parenteral, and carefully monitoring the patient for seemingly small changes.

Measuring Outcome Indicators

Outcome indicators may be pre-established, such as helping a client reduce cholesterol levels to under 200 mg/dL, a common benchmark for cholesterol. Outcome indicators may also vary by individual circumstance, such as helping a client with an eating disorder gain weight. Collecting baseline data, documenting the intervention, and collecting post-intervention data relevant to the desired outcome is a comprehensive way to measure outcomes.

Nutrition evaluation measures objective outcomes to determine whether the patient's health and behavior has improved as a result of the care plan and if the nutrition plan is successful.

Indicators

Indicators help to determine which processes and outcomes may require more attention to assure the quality of the care plan, which allows the nutrition professional to make adjustments to the program if necessary.

Rate-based indicators evaluate what the outcome may be if the best possible care is provided, expressed as a rate or proportion. An indicator will determine a tolerable best-case outcome, and if this outcome is not met, re-evaluation will be required.

Sentinel event indicators are serious events or incidents that make it necessary to further investigate the care plan. The threshold for these indicators is always 0 percent or 100 percent.

Evaluating Outcomes for Common Conditions

Direct Nutrition Outcomes

These outcomes are usually collected when a nutrient deficiency (and perhaps a related disease) are present. These outcomes relate to the presence of micronutrient and macronutrient diversity and consumption in an individual's diet. A client experiencing side affects of anemia, such as dizziness or fainting, may be prescribed an oral iron supplement. Blood testing and monitoring can show whether iron supplementation is helping the client.

Clinical and Health Status Outcomes

These outcomes are usually collected when a client's chronic health problem, such as cardiovascular disease or obesity, are being addressed. These outcomes relate to changes in the client's anthropometric and/or biochemical measurements. For example, a client with borderline-high cholesterol levels may be advised to adopt a more plant-based diet, limiting foods that are higher in cholesterol. Regular cholesterol testing after this modification can show whether or not it is producing the desired outcome.

Patient-Centered Outcomes

These outcomes are usually collected when the client has a specific concern he or she would like to address; normally, they are voluntarily seeking treatment. These outcomes relate to measurements that are important to the patient, though they may not always be medically necessary. For example, a client may want to understand if dietary changes can help him or her sleep better at night; in this case, the practitioner may recommend eliminating caffeine, sugar, and alcohol in afternoons and evenings. Or, a client may be training for a vigorous event such as an obstacle race or triathlon. In this situation, he or she may want some guidance on how to eat each day for the most effective training. In both of these contexts, nutritional guidance is not directly a matter of life or death; rather, it is sought in order to reach an outcome that the client desires.

Healthcare Utilization Outcomes

These outcomes are usually collected around how clients utilize their health care resources, such as seeking nutritional guidance if their health insurance covers it. They can also focus on how clients sustain outcomes achieved from their treatment over time.

Evaluating Learner Knowledge and Performance

These outcomes are usually collected when treatment includes an educational component, such as diet counseling for non-surgical bariatric patients and any health changes that occur after the treatment. They are often evaluated using pre- and post-tests.

Communicating with Dietitian

Dietetic technicians work closely with dietitians. Communication regarding a client may occur face-to-face, over email, through an electronic medical record, or through paper charting. A dietetic technician may work alongside the dietitian during a client session. In busy practices, dietitians may rely heavily on dietetic technicians in order to meet the needs of the high volume of patients; therefore, it is vital to follow good documentation practices, detailed recordkeeping methods, and maintain a close, positive working relationship.

Documentation

Privacy of Medical Information (e.g., HIPAA)
HIPAA
HIPAA stands for Health Insurance Portability and Accountability Act. It was implemented in 1996 and is also known as the Kenned-Kassebaum Act. Essentially, HIPAA is a set of guidelines that should be followed when preparing medical documentation, due to the fact that it is a permanent legal document. The four main objectives are to regulate sharing of information via computers, provide universal identifiers for healthcare providers and plans, implement information security regulations, and establish a privacy rule. The privacy rule is particularly important to nutrition professionals because it outlines how medical information should be handled. Also, all notes should be written in black ink or typed and entries should be made during or immediately following the patient's visit and should be signed and dated. A nutrition professional should contact the doctor who prescribed the diet order if they suspect it is incorrect, rather than changing the note themselves. If a note is changed, a single line should be drawn through the mistake and then initialed and dated.

Privacy Rule
The privacy rule was established in 2003 to address the patients' right to privacy regarding their medical care. All patients receive this privacy notice at their initial visit to a health care provider. The patient's medical record must also be kept confidential. The medical team, the patient, and their designated representative should be the only people with access to the information in the medical chart.

Data Mining
Data mining utilizes software algorithms to examine large datasets and find trends. Practitioners may record certain pieces of data from client interactions, such as nutrient counts from the client's food log, and record them into a database. From there, dietary patterns or indicators can emerge related to the client's health status or health goals.

Healthcare Informatics and Technologies

Healthcare informatics and technologies have replaced most traditional paper methods of collecting and storing information.

Electronic Medical Record
Another critical aspect of client management is the maintenance of the case records. All documentation is typically added to an electronic health record (EHR), also called electronic medical records (EMR), due to the need to maintain patient privacy and confidentiality. The use of paper records continues, but due to the volume of information collected and the need to ensure the security of these records, this practice will soon be phased out. Basic standards of care require the EHR contains all pertinent information and that it is updated frequently as the plan of care changes. Basic demographic information, along with treatment protocols and correspondence, is readily available to be accessed by

the necessary practitioners associated with the case. Further, the meaningful use of the file sharing is expected. Meaning, one of the main stipulations of the use of the EHR is that the client and provider benefit from the use of the EHR in quantifiable and qualitative ways. For this reason, it is imperative nutrition professionals address the client's progress throughout the treatment plan in the EHR.

Nutrient Analysis and Databases
National Nutrient Database for Standard Reference is available at the following web address: https://ndb.nal.usda.gov/. It contains nutrient information on almost 9,000 foods and is maintained by the Nutrient Data Laboratory. Special interest databases include Flavonoids, Isoflavones, and Proanthocyanidins.

Everything Added to Food in the United States (EAFUS) is available at the following web address http://www.fda.gov/Food/IngredientsPackagingLabeling/FoodAdditivesIngredients/ucm115326.htm. The database is maintained by the U.S. Food and Drug Administration Center for Food Safety and Applied Nutrition (CFSAN) under the Priority-based Assessment of Food Additives (PAFA) program. PAFA contains information on over 2,000 substances added to food that the FDA has either approved as a food additive or listed as Generally Regarded As Safe (GRAS). This is not an exhaustive list, as some ingredients added to food are not regulated by the FDA.

The Ground Beef Calculator allows the user to view nutrient information for raw or cooked beef based on either fat or lean percentage.

Regulations for Nutrition Labels
The FDA is currently updating its requirements for nutrition labels. As of 2013, nutrition labels should be placed near the product's ingredient list and manufacturing information. Serving size, number of servings, and calories are listed near the top of the label. Vitamin A, vitamin C, calcium, iron, enrichment vitamins, total fat, total carbohydrate, total protein, total sodium, calories from fat, saturated fat, trans fat, cholesterol, and sugar are also included; percent of daily value of each component must be listed. Foods that are exempt from nutrition labeling requirements include infant formula, direct-to-consumer deli, bakery, and restaurant products, dietary supplements, bulk foods, fresh produce, fresh seafood, and foods without nutritional value.

Components of the Intake Domain in Nutrition Diagnostic Labeling
The intake domain of the nutrition diagnosis includes complications that involve the intake of energy, nutrients, and fluids, regardless of what type of nutrition the patient receives, including oral, enteral, or parenteral nutrition. There are five classes included within the intake domain: calorie energy balance, oral or nutrition support intake, fluid intake balance, bioactive substance charting, and nutrient balance.

- *Calorie energy balance* is a description of observed or potential changes in energy expenditure. These changes can be due to conditions such as anorexia, dialysis, trauma, or any other diagnosis that disrupts the catabolic or anabolic state.

- *Oral or nutrition support intake* refers to adequate or excessive intake compared to the goal.

- *Fluid intake balance* is also described as adequate or excessive intake compared to the goal. This is significant in diseases where fluid intake needs to be closely monitored or restricted, such as kidney disease.

- *Bioactive substance charting* is the area where the dietitian can note miscellaneous substances ingested by the patients such as supplements, multivitamins, or alcohol.

- *Nutrient balance* expands on the bioactive substance chart aspect. Use of vitamin or mineral supplements can lead to excessive intake of a single nutrient.

Behavioral-Environmental Domain in Nutrition Diagnostic Labeling

The behavioral-environmental domain refers to problems or concerns involving the patient's knowledge, attitudes, beliefs, environmental factors, food safety, and ability to access food due to financial or transportation issues. All of these factors can contribute to an individual's nutritional status. Long-held cultural practices may put an individual at a nutritional risk. For example, The Native American tradition of feeding infants sugar-sweetened drinks will eventually lead to tooth decay in young children. The physical activity balance of this domain may refer to an elderly individual who can no longer travel to purchase healthy foods or loses the ability to prepare meals. Another example of this class would be a highly sedentary individual whose inactivity puts them at an increased risk of obesity or disease that can be a result of obesity. Food safety refers to an individual's ability to safely store and prepare foods. For example, a homeless person will not be able to refrigerate foods or bring them to a proper temperature during the cooking process, leading to the risk of foods sitting in the temperature danger zone and causing a foodborne illness.

PESS Statement

Within the nutrition diagnosis, the dietitian should utilize the PESS format when describing the issue. This is a standardized method that includes the problem, etiology, signs, and symptoms (PESS). The PESS statement can be written using language pulled from the International Dietetic and Nutrition Terminology (IDNT) Reference Manual, which breaks down each part of the statement using standardized language. The first part of the PESS statement is the problem, which must be an approved diagnostic label and include an adjective that describes how the patient's issue differs from what would be the desired state of health. Examples of a problem within a PESS statement could include: "altered mental status," "impaired bowel syndrome," "chronic renal failure," or "at risk of liver cirrhosis." The next part of this statement is the etiology, which describes the cause or the problem or factors contributing to the problem. These may be physical, situational, cultural, developmental, or anything that may be an underlying cause of the problem. The last part of the PESS statement describes the signs and symptoms of the condition being described including physical symptoms or data from lab tests and anthropometric tests. The PESS statement must be written in a specific way: the Problem "related to" Etiology "as evidenced by" Signs and Symptoms.

Evaluation of Education Programs

Implementation

Implementing an education program requires determining the duration, frequency, and intensity of educational sessions. Facilitators should ensure that participants feel comfortable attending and engaging during sessions. Sessions should be consistent, reliable in nature, and include program feedback from the participants.

Communication

Interpersonal

This form of communication occurs between two or more people who are somewhat familiar with one another (such as students and teachers, a group of friends, or spouses). It can be face-to-face or through another medium. This form of communication takes into consideration both verbal and non-verbal cues. It is primarily used to foster and nurture relationships.

Group Process

This form of communication refers to how groups interact in order to complete a task. Normally, the group has a common goal, but they may not know anything else about one another. The group process focuses on how individuals cooperate in order to achieve their common purpose, resolve conflicts, make decisions, and document results.

Methods of Instruction

Instruction can be facilitated, interactive, teacher-led, or student-led. It can involve handouts, exercises, tasks, and ongoing assignments that focus on the topic of instruction. Technological tools such as slideshows, videos, virtual classrooms, and social media can also be utilized.

Evaluation of Educational Outcomes

Formative

Formative evaluation can take place at any point during the program. They are usually focused on continuous improvement; these evaluations note processes that are in place and evaluate how they are working, and how they can be improved. Formative evaluations are important components of pilot programs. However, they can also be used in established programs to examine progress at periods of time (such as quarterly benchmarks).

Summative

Summative evaluations focus on outcomes achieved rather than processes in place. They evaluate whether the pre-established outcome was achieved as a result of the program. These occur at the end of the intervention, rather than during.

Evaluating the Effectiveness of Educational Plans

Formative and summative evaluations are important components in determining whether or not a program is effective overall. Together, they examine the constructs that make up the program as well as the outcomes that should result. This overall evaluation is an important tool in engaging key stakeholders, maintaining funding, addressing opportunities for improvement, and contributing to future research and educational efforts.

Practice Questions

1. Which of the following is appropriate to include in the physical assessment of a new patient?
   a. Height
   b. Weight history
   c. Food preferences
   d. Both A and B

2. When making diet recommendations, which part of the clinical assessment is the most important?
   a. Physical assessment
   b. Psychosocial assessment
   c. Biochemical test results
   d. All of the above

3. What program seeks to assess how well-existing programs are serving the health needs of the community?
   a. Nutritional Assessment of Populations
   b. Women, Infant, Children Program
   c. Supplemental Nutrition Assistance Program
   d. National Dietary Surveillance

4. What populations have experienced a particularly large increase in the rate of diabetes due to diet changes?
   a. Native American
   b. Alaskan Native
   c. Pacific Islander
   d. Both A and B

5. Which of the following could be administered during a patient interview to assist with obtaining a diet history?
   a. Three-day food record ✗
   b. Food frequency questionnaire
   c. Motivational interviewing ✗
   d. Twenty-four-hour recall

6. What is one of the programs managed by the CDC to monitor the health and nutritional status of low-income women, infants, and children?
   a. PedNSS
   b. WIC
   c. NSS
   d. EPSDT

7. Poorly treated diabetes can have many adverse outcomes including which of the following?
   a. Weight gain
   b. Weight loss
   c. Blindness
   d. Anorexia

8. In diabetes, which of the following is true regarding glucose?
    a. It is unable to reach the cells.
    b. It is poorly absorbed.
    c. It is absorbed too quickly.
    d. It is not broken down.

9. Which statement represents part of the nutritional therapy for an individual with Type 2 diabetes?
    a. Decrease caloric intake
    b. Decrease the number of snacks consumed daily
    c. Do not eat after 9 p.m.
    d. Keep carbohydrate intake consistent during the day

10. A woman who is 5'6" tall and weighs 130 pounds has a BMI in which range?
    a. Healthy range
    b. Underweight range
    c. Overweight range
    d. Obese range

11. You read in a patient's medical record that she has Type 1 diabetes and does not have a regular dietary intake. What advice should she be given?
    a. Keep this eating plan if she is not overweight.
    b. Start eating regularly scheduled meals and snacks, and insulin dosing is based on meal pattern.
    c. No additional advice is needed.
    d. Ask her to record her blood sugar levels.

12. Which section of the intestine is most likely involved in Crohn's disease?
    a. Colon
    b. Ileum
    c. Jejunum
    d. Duodenum

13. You are performing a diet assessment on a child recently diagnosed with AIDS. The diet should consist of which of the following?
    a. High fat and high protein
    b. High protein and high in vitamins and minerals
    c. High calorie and high protein
    d. High protein and high fluids

14. Which of the following puts a woman at an increased risk of gestational diabetes?
    a. If she has a history of gestational diabetes.
    b. If she has a pre-pregnancy BMI greater than 26.
    c. If she is over the age of thirty-five.
    d. If she conceived within ten months of a previous pregnancy.

15. A baby born to a mother with gestational diabetes is at increased risk for which of the following?
    a. Fetal hypoglycemia at birth
    b. Fetal macrosomia
    c. Fetal macrocephaly
    d. Both A and B

16. You are working with an individual who is newly diagnosed with Type 2 diabetes. What advice would you give regarding lipid levels?
    a. HDL levels should be above 40
    b. LDL levels should be below 110
    c. TG levels should be below 100
    d. Total cholesterol should be below 150

17. Which of the following are symptoms of renal disease?
    a. Weight loss, anorexia, vomiting
    b. Fever, weight gain, anorexia
    c. Anorexia, weight loss, edema
    d. Edema, anemia, vomiting

18. Which range represents the appropriate amount of potassium a patient with chronic renal failure on hemodialysis should consume on a daily basis?
    a. 2 to 4 grams
    b. 2 to 3 grams
    c. 1 to 2 grams
    d. 3 to 4 grams

19. A person who must avoid milk and all dairy products might be deficient in which nutrients?
    a. Protein, calories✗
    b. Calcium, vitamin A
    c. Vitamin D, calcium
    d. Vitamin B12, vitamin D✗

20. Which of the following is advice that should be given to an individual with Crohn's disease?
    a. Decrease fiber, increase intake of fat soluble vitamins
    b. Decrease fat intake, increase fiber intake
    c. Supplement with vitamin C and vitamin B12
    d. Increase protein intake, supplement vitamin D

21. A product containing which of the following would not be suitable for a person with a milk protein allergy?
    a. Lactose
    b. Whey
    c. Calcium
    d. All of the above are safe in milk allergy

22. Which of the following is appropriate for an individual with Celiac disease?
    a. Beer
    b. Rye bread
    c. Potato bread
    d. White bread

23. What mineral has been shown to help provide protective benefits against cancer?
    a. Vitamin C
    b. Vitamin D
    c. Vitamin A
    d. Vitamin K

24. A patient with cancer would like some advice on how to cook foods during her chemotherapy treatment. Which of the following is appropriate advice?
   a. There is no need to change how you cook your food.
   b. Utilize moist heat cooking methods to keep your meats tender.
   c. Check to ensure all foods are cooked to the correct temperature.
   d. Avoid using large quantities of salt.

25. Current recommendations suggest that individuals with heart disease should consume less than how many milligrams of cholesterol per day?
   a. 300
   b. 200
   c. 250
   d. 325

26. Which diet pattern emphasizes whole grains, fruits, vegetables, fish, healthy fats, and low-fat dairy?
   a. NASH
   b. DASH
   c. Atkins
   d. South Beach

27. Which of the following products could you recommend to a pregnant woman who would like to increase her daily intake of folic acid?
   a. Organic pasta
   b. Organic wheat bread
   c. Black beans
   d. Eggs

28. The spouse of an individual recently diagnosed with Alzheimer's disease is concerned about recent decreased oral intake. What could you recommend to help improve oral intake?
   a. Eat in front of the TV.
   b. Try to stick to a regular meal schedule.
   c. Eat with other people as often as possible.
   d. Encourage the spouse to pick his/her own foods.

29. Which of the following is a symptom of dehydration?
   a. Confusion
   b. Light-headedness
   c. Dizziness
   d. All of the above

30. Which foods could you recommend to someone with iron deficiency anemia?
   a. Dried fruit, dried peas and beans, eggs
   b. Beef, dried fruit, dried peas and beans
   c. Milk, eggs, liver
   d. Fortified whole grain pasta, cheese

31. You work at an assisted living facility and are conducting a physical exam on a new resident. What is a warning sign of malnutrition?
   a. Extended history of a BMI of 20
   b. Poorly fitting dentures
   c. A stage 1 pressure ulcer
   d. Recent bout of confusion

32. A patient was just admitted to your unit with a diagnosis of anorexia nervosa. What is one of the immediate concerns with this patient?
   a. Increase calorie needs by approximately 100 to 300 calories
   b. Increase fluid intake
   c. Place consult request with the inpatient behavioral therapist
   d. Correct electrolyte balance

33. Which of the following could be signs of bulimia?
   a. Advanced tooth decay, distended abdomen
   b. Throat inflammation, advanced tooth decay
   c. Epigastric pain, Throat inflammation
   d. Edema, Epigastric pain

34. A patient with a gastric ulcer currently on medication therapy is asking for diet advice. Which of the following is the most prudent?
   a. Drink milk to help coat the stomach.
   b. Avoid excess caffeine and alcohol.
   c. Eat a low fat diet.
   d. Eat a high fiber diet.

35. Dumping syndrome occurs when large amounts of partially digested food pass into what structure?
   a. Ileum
   b. Duodenum
   c. Jejunum
   d. Colon

36. Dumping syndrome can occur when?
   a. In individuals who have had a gastrectomy
   b. In dehydrated individuals
   c. In individuals that consume a high carbohydrate diet
   d. A and C

37. A person with diverticulosis not experiencing a flare in symptoms should follow which type of diet?
   a. High fiber
   b. Low fiber
   c. Low fat
   d. Low residue

38. You are conducting a nutrition screening on a patient admitted for sustained, abnormally low blood pressure. They mention that they are concerned about a recent bout with diverticulitis. What type of diet would you recommend?
    a. Low fat
    b. Low fiber
    c. Elemental
    d. Clear liquids only

39. Someone living with Crohn's disease may be anemic due to which of the following?
    a. Intake of only non-heme sources of iron
    b. Blood loss and poor absorption
    c. A and B
    d. High intake of calcium

40. During an acute flare of Crohn's disease, medical treatment consists of which of the following?
    a. TPN
    b. Elemental diet
    c. Maintenance of fluid and electrolyte balance
    d. Complete bowel rest

41. A poorly controlled asthmatic has been admitted to the hospital with an acute asthma flare. You note a long history of prednisone use. Which nutrients may be at risk for deficiency?
    a. Calcium, Vitamin D
    b. Vitamin D
    c. Phosphorus
    d. Not enough information to answer the question

42. What is steatorrhea?
    a. The presence of protein in the stool
    b. The presence of fat in the stool
    c. Large, soft stools
    d. Small, frequent stooling

43. When does Short Bowel Syndrome occur?
    a. A baby is born without all of its intestine fully developed
    b. Significant sections of the small intestine have been removed
    c. Significant sections of the large intestine have been removed
    d. The intestine loses its ability to fully absorb nutrients

44. What vitamins and minerals may need to be supplemented in an individual following intestinal resection?
    a. Vitamin D, Vitamin C, Zinc
    b. Vitamin B12, Iron, Zinc, Vitamin B6
    c. Vitamin B12, Calcium, Iron, Zinc
    d. Calcium, Vitamin B6, Zinc

45. What is best form of nutrition for a patient following a bowel resection surgery?
   a. TPN
   b. EN
   c. Elemental diet
   d. Regular oral diet as tolerated

46. Liver failure is defined as the function of the liver being reduced to what percentage or less?
   a. 35%
   b. 40%
   c. 25%
   d. 30%

47. A patient with liver disease has followed the advice of the dietitian and primarily uses medium train triglycerides (MCT) as a fat source. What needs to be supplemented in order to avoid an essential fatty acid deficiency?
   a. Linolenic acid
   b. Linoleic acid
   c. DHA
   d. EPA

48. The liver is the primary source of alcohol metabolism. Alcohol metabolism requires what vitamins?
   a. Fat soluble vitamins
   b. Water soluble vitamins
   c. B vitamins
   d. Vitamin B12 and Vitamin D

49. In cirrhosis, blood flow around the liver is disrupted by what?
   a. Muscle fibers tissue
   b. Nonfunctional connective tissue
   c. Ascites
   d. Edema

50. What is the function of the gall bladder?
   a. Filter toxic elements
   b. Metabolize and store nutrients
   c. Regulate fluid and electrolyte balance
   d. Concentrate and store bile

51. Cholecystitis is inflammation of which of the following?
   a. The liver, which causes excess water to be absorbed, allowing cholesterol to precipitate out, which causes cholelithiasis
   b. The gallbladder, which causes excess water to be absorbed, allowing cholesterol to precipitate out, which causes cholelithiasis
   c. The colon, which causes excess water to be absorbed, allowing cholesterol to precipitate out, which causes cholelithiasis
   d. None of the above

52. Which of the following is a symptom of acute pancreatitis?
    a. Weight loss
    b. Steatorrhea
    c. Severe abdominal pain
    d. Malabsorption of fat soluble vitamins

53. Which of the following describes an appropriate diet for someone with cystic fibrosis?
    a. High calorie, high protein, unrestricted fat, high salt
    b. High protein, moderate fat, moderate salt
    c. High calorie, moderate protein and fat, high salt
    d. Unrestricted fat, moderate protein, low salt

54. Why does fluid intake sometimes need to be restricted in a patient with congestive heart failure?
    a. The heart pumps more slowly, causing fluid to be held in the tissues.
    b. The body retains more sodium, causing fluid to be retained.
    c. The heart pumps less efficiently, causing fluid to be held in the tissues.
    d. The kidneys no longer filter sodium, causing fluid to be retained.

55. Gout can result in excessive levels of what in the blood?
    a. Uric acid
    b. Ammonia
    c. Nitrogen
    d. Creatinine

56. An endemic goiter occurs in which of the following cases?
    a. An individual who has an enlargement of the thyroid gland due to insufficient thyroid hormone
    b. An individual who consumes a diet low in iodine
    c. An individual who is taking levothyroxine
    d. None of the above

57. Anticonvulsants used to treat epilepsy interfere with the absorption of what mineral?
    a. Zinc
    b. Magnesium
    c. Calcium
    d. Riboflavin

58. What is anaphylaxis?
    a. A severe reaction to a food
    b. A severe reaction to a medicine
    c. A severe reaction to a micronutrient
    d. Both A and B

59. Which of the following is not considered to be one of the top allergenic foods?
    a. Peanuts
    b. Milk
    c. Sesame
    d. Eggs

60. Initial treatment of a burn patient should focus on which of the following?
    a. Replacing fluids and electrolytes
    b. Increasing protein intake to promote wound healing
    c. Supplementation of vitamin C and zinc to promote wound healing
    d. Providing adequate calories to prevent ketosis

61. Aspirin can interfere with the absorption of which of the following?
    a. Vitamin D
    b. Ascorbic Acid
    c. Alpha-tocopherol
    d. Calcium

62. Corticosteroids can cause which of the following?
    a. A decrease in calcium absorption and protein synthesis
    b. An increase in calcium absorption and protein synthesis
    c. A decrease in calcium absorption and increase in protein synthesis
    d. An increase in calcium absorption and decrease in protein synthesis

63. Diarrhea can quickly deplete the body's stores of what?
    a. Sodium, Magnesium
    b. Magnesium, Potassium
    c. Sodium, Potassium
    d. Sodium, Magnesium, Potassium

64. Current guidelines suggest that patients recovering from surgery should wait how long to begin oral feeding?
    a. 24 to 48 hours
    b. 12 to 24 hours
    c. 24 to 36 hours
    d. 6 to 12 hours

65. A patient experiencing a delay in nutrition support following an injury is at an increased risk for which of the following?
    a. Poor wound healing
    b. Lower immune system function
    c. Albumin depletion
    d. All of the above

66. You calculate a patient's BMI as 26.8 kg/m^2. How would you categorize this patient?
    a. Underweight
    b. Overweight
    c. Healthy weight
    d. Obese

67. An otherwise healthy adult asks you for some advice on how to modify their lifestyle and diet to begin to lose weight. You recommend reducing daily caloric intake by how many calories to encourage losing approximately 1 pound of weight per week?
    a. 500 calories
    b. 550 calories
    c. 400 calories
    d. 450 calories

68. What is the mechanism that could possibly explain why patients undergoing chemotherapy treatment may experience more frequent nausea and vomiting?
    a. The route by which the medication is administered
    b. The speed at which the medication is administered
    c. The medication targets rapidly dividing cells, which can influence the cells of the GI tract
    d. The medication targets the stomach mucosa, leading to increased inflammation

69. Which scenario favors the formation of dental caries?
    a. Eating a large portion of dessert
    b. Snacking throughout the day
    c. Eating shortly before going to bed
    d. Eating highly acidic foods

70. Which of the following is one of the primary goals of nutritional therapy in AIDS patients?
    a. Find sources of unsaturated fatty acids
    b. Increase fluid intake
    c. Prevent protein malnutrition
    d. Supplement with fat-soluble vitamins

71. Breastfeeding is contraindicated for which of the following mothers?
    a. A mom with a Strep infection on amoxicillin
    b. A mom with a cold not currently taking any medications for symptoms
    c. A mom with severe allergies currently taking Zyrtec
    d. A mom with HIV

72. You are conducting an assessment on a patient with long standing COPD. After you finish the physical and psychosocial assessments, and review biochemical labs, you become concerned that the patient may be in early stages of protein-energy malnutrition. What could be the culprit?
    a. Increased energy demands of COPD
    b. The patient eats a diet high in carbohydrates
    c. The patient prefers to eat small meals during the day
    d. All of the above

73. In nutrition diagnostic labeling, problems that can be physical or mechanical and interfere with one's ability to achieve normal nutrition status are known as which of the following?
    a. Functional balance
    b. Biochemical balance
    c. Weight balance
    d. None of the above

74. In nutrition diagnostic labeling, which of the following indicates a loss of the ability to normally metabolize foods due to medication intake, surgery, or a disease process?
    a. Functional balance
    b. Biochemical balance
    c. Weight balance
    d. None of the above

75. In nutrition diagnostic labeling, which of the following describes the involuntary weight changes that can cause a patient to deviate from the patient's normal or desired body weight?
    a. Functional balance
    b. Biochemical balance
    c. Weight balance
    d. None of the above

76. The components of the intake domain in nutrition diagnostic labeling contain all but which of the following pieces of information?
    a. Energy intake
    b. Patient's knowledge about food
    c. Fluid intake
    d. Vitamin/Mineral intake

77. The intake domain in nutrition diagnostic labeling contains five classes of concern. Which of the following is not one of those five classes?
    a. Patient access to food
    b. Nutrient balance
    c. Fluid intake
    d. Oral intake

78. Which of the following is not part of the behavioral-environmental domain in nutrition diagnostic labeling?
    a. Patient's knowledge of food safety
    b. Patient's access to food
    c. Patient's attitudes about food
    d. Patient's nutrient balance

79. Which of the following represents an accurate PES statement?
    a. Altered mental status related to dementia caused by dehydration
    b. Altered mental status of dementia due to decreased fluid intake
    c. Altered mental status related to dehydration as evidenced by biochemical labs
    d. Altered mental status related to dehydration due to decreased fluid intake

80. A dietitian may ask for your assistance on educating a newly diagnosed patient with congestive heart failure about a heart healthy diet. A diet specifically tailored to a patient's needs is called what?
    a. Therapeutic
    b. Lifestyle change
    c. DASH diet
    d. Mediterranean diet

81. You have been asked to provide a diet education for a patient about to be discharged. The patient was hospitalized with protein-energy malnutrition. What type of diet should the patient follow to help reduce the risk of developing protein-energy malnutrition again?
    a. Vegetarian
    b. Kosher
    c. High Protein
    d. High calorie, high protein

82. Which of the following items would not be acceptable to recommend for a patient following a lacto-vegetarian eating pattern?
    a. Cheese
    b. Yogurt
    c. Eggs
    d. Tofu

83. Which diet is very low in carbohydrate and high in fat to help treat seizure disorders?
    a. High calorie, high protein
    b. Ketogenic
    c. Vegetarian
    d. Galactosemic

84. The hemodialysis diet restricts which of the following nutrients?
    a. Sodium
    b. Sodium, Phosphorus
    c. Sodium, Phosphorus, Potassium
    d. Sodium, Phosphorus, Potassium, Magnesium

85. If an individual diagnosed with hypertension is truly salt sensitive, how much sodium should their diet contain?
    a. 1,300 mg or less
    b. 1,500 mg or less
    c. 1,700 mg or less
    d. 1,900 mg or less

86. A child was recently diagnosed with galactosemia. The parents should be instructed that life-long avoidance of which of the following foods is required to prevent complications?
    a. Milk
    b. Kiwi
    c. Avocado
    d. Beef

87. How often should formula used in an enteral feeding system be discarded to avoid bacterial contamination?
    a. Every 6 hours
    b. Every 12 hours
    c. Every 18 hours
    d. Every 24 hours

88. Which of the following patients is the most appropriate for enteral feeding?
    a. A 90-year-old female recovering from hip surgery
    b. A 25-year-old male recovering from oral surgery
    c. A 45-year-old female recovering from bowel resection
    d. A 65-year-old male with dysphagia to thin liquids

89. When does refeeding syndrome occur?
    a. Potassium rapidly leaves the plasma and enters the cells to become a part of adenosine triphosphate
    b. Phosphorus rapidly leaves the plasma and enters the cells to become a part of adenosine triphosphate
    c. Glucose rapidly leaves the plasma and enters the cells to become a part of adenosine triphosphate
    d. Phosphate rapidly leaves the plasma and enters the cells to become a part of adenosine triphosphate

90. Which patient is at an increased risk for developing refeeding syndrome?
    a. An alcoholic who frequently fasts for several days while on drinking binges
    b. An athlete who is attempting to lose five pounds in five days
    c. An anorexic currently in recovery
    d. A patient currently on TPN

91. According to the Adult Treatment Panel III Report, which of the following individuals is at an increased risk for heart disease with a LDL level about 100?
    a. A 35-year-old male with diabetes
    b. A 65-year-old male without any underlying conditions
    c. A 40-year-old female with a BMI over 30
    d. A 55-year-old female that consumes a high fat diet

92. The Adult Treatment Panel III Report recommends which of the following therapeutic lifestyle changes to help reduce LDL levels and therefore reduce the risk of developing heart disease?
    a. Decrease sodium intake
    b. Decrease intake of unsaturated fatty acids
    c. Increase fiber intake
    d. Consume no more than 300 mg/day of cholesterol

93. Which of the following was developed to give dietitians a common structure and method to promote better decision-making and to obtain data that may be evaluated quantitatively and qualitatively?
    a. Nutrition Screening Process
    b. Nutrition Therapy Process
    c. Nutrition Care Process
    d. Nutrition Care Protocol

94. Which of the following is not a USDA program?
    a. National School Lunch Program
    b. WIC
    c. Supplemental Nutrition Assistance Program
    d. Food Banks

95. A patient was discharged from the hospital on a high calorie, high protein diet. The following statements were included in the nutrition note during a one-month follow-up. Which one belongs in the evaluation section of the note?

    a. Patient states no changes in appetite since discharge from the hospital.

    b. Patient has gained approximately 1 kg since discharge, meeting initial nutrition goal.

    c. Patient is getting assistance from a home health company in preparing meals.

    d. Patient states she enjoys cooking again.

96. Which of the following is considered protected health information under HIPAA guidelines?

    a. Patient gender

    b. Patient diagnosis

    c. Patient date of birth

    d. Patient hospital discharge date

97. What substance, found in beef, contributes to its color?

    a. Myoglobin

    b. Collagen

    c. Fibrils

    d. Amino Acids

98. What function do eggs serve in baked goods?

    a. Structure

    b. Color

    c. Protein

    d. All of the above

99. What source of protein is considered very high quality because it contains all of the amino acids essential to the human body?

    a. Beef

    b. Chicken

    c. Fish

    d. Eggs

100. Which type of pasteurization extends shelf life of milk?

    a. Ultra-High Temperature

    b. Cold Pasteurization

    c. High Temperature Pasteurization

    d. Flash Pasteurization

101. Evaporated milk has had what percent of water removed?

    a. 75%

    b. 15%

    c. 60%

    d. 50%

102. Low lactose milk is treated with which of the following?

    a. Lactase

    b. Maltase

    c. Sucrase

    d. Fructase

103. Which gas is naturally given off by fruits and is responsible for ripening?
   a. Methane
   b. Ethylene
   c. Nitrogen
   d. Oxygen

104. Which phytochemical is least affected by the pH of a cooking solution?
   a. Isoflavone
   b. Chlorophyll
   c. Carotenoids
   d. Lycopenes

105. Which phytochemical is an antioxidant and protects against conditions such as heart disease?
   a. Lycopene
   b. Chlorophyll
   c. Anthocynanins
   d. Chlorophyll

106. What chemical reaction takes place as fruit ripens?
   a. Pectin is broken down by pectic acid.
   b. Starch is converted to sugar.
   c. Hemicellulose is broken down to cellulose.
   d. Enzymes soften lignin.

107. Which of the following lists the protein content of flour from least to greatest?
   a. All purpose, Cake, Pastry, Bread
   b. Bread, All purpose, Cake, Pastry
   c. All purpose, Pastry, Bread, Cake
   d. Cake, Pastry, All purpose, Bread

108. Gluten provides all but which of the following functions?
   a. Structure
   b. Elastic properties
   c. Color
   d. Holds leavening agents

109. Adding fat to baked products contributes to which of the following characteristics?
   a. Color
   b. Tenderness
   c. Structure
   d. Elastic properties

110. Which of the following best explains how engineered foods or genetically engineered food is made?
   a. Inserting genes from one organism into another
   b. Allowing plants to cross breed with one another
   c. Inserting genes from one plant to another plant
   d. Using bacteria to alter the genetic make-up of organisms

111. Yogurt can be considered what type of food?
    a. Engineered
    b. Functional
    c. Fortified
    d. Homogenized

112. Dry heat cooking methods are best suited for which of the following?
    a. Cuts of meat with a high fat content
    b. Aged cuts of meat
    c. Cuts of meat with less connective tissue
    d. Cuts of meat with more connective tissue

113. Which of the following are moist heat cooking methods?
    a. Frying
    b. Braising
    c. Stewing
    d. Both B and C

114. Nitrates and Nitrites, additives used in processed meats, serve what function?
    a. Contribute to flavor
    b. Extend shelf life
    c. Inhibit the growth of C. botulinum
    d. Enhance color

115. Carbohydrates contribute how many kilocalories per gram?
    a. 4 kilocalories
    b. 5 kilocalories
    c. 7 kilocalories
    d. 9 kilocalories

116. Protein contributes how many kilocalories per gram?
    a. 4 kilocalories
    b. 5 kilocalories
    c. 7 kilocalories
    d. 9 kilocalories

117. Fat contributes how many kilocalories per gram?
    a. 4 kilocalories
    b. 5 kilocalories
    c. 7 kilocalories
    d. 9 kilocalories

118. What is one of the most abundant sources of carbohydrates in the diet?
    a. Fruits
    b. Vegetables
    c. Starch
    d. Fiber

119. Good sources of which type of fatty acids include fish, ground flax seeds, walnuts, canola oil, and soybean oil.
    a. Omega 3
    b. Omega 6
    c. Omega 9
    d. Omega 12

120. Which of the following is/are needed in large quantities in order to provide the body what it needs to maintain a healthy immune system?
    a. Micronutrients
    b. Zinc
    c. Iodine
    d. Macronutrients

121. What organization maintains the National Nutrient Database for Standard Reference?
    a. USDA
    b. FDA
    c. National Data Laboratory
    d. Nutrient Data Laboratory

122. Which of the following is the correct list of macronutrients?
    a. Carbohydrates, Fat, Protein, Minerals
    b. Carbohydrates, Fat, Protein, Vitamins, Minerals
    c. Carbohydrates, Fat, Protein
    d. Carbohydrates, Fat, Protein, Phytochemicals, Vitamins Minerals

123. What is the preferred substrate for the brain?
    a. Lipids
    b. Amino Acids
    c. Glucose
    d. Unsaturated fatty acids

124. Which of the following is an important physiological process breaking down macro- and micro-nutrients into smaller, more easily absorbed forms that can be utilized by the body?
    a. Digestion
    b. Ingestion
    c. Absorption
    d. Circulation

125. Which of the following hormones does not regulates digestion?
    a. CCK
    b. Insulin
    c. Gastrin
    d. Secretic

126. The metabolic rate is influenced by which of the following?
    a. Hormonal status, age, gender, rate of digestion
    b. Body size and composition, age, gender, and hormonal status
    c. Gender, weight, age, hormonal status, body composition
    d. Body size and composition, absorptive capacity, hormonal status, age

127. Which organ helps the body excrete waste?
    a. Stomach
    b. Heart
    c. Lungs
    d. Liver

128. Which left stage requires the greatest number of calories and protein per kg of body weight?
    a. Adolescence
    b. Geriatric
    c. Infancy
    d. Childhood

129. In what life stage(s) is growth most rapid in normally developing children?
    a. Infancy and Childhood
    b. Infancy and Adolescence
    c. Infancy
    d. Adolescence

130. An adult asks you for assistance with their diet. They are free from chronic disease and do not have any other underlying conditions that give them specific nutrient needs. What percentage of their total caloric intake should come from carbohydrates?
    a. 15% to 25%
    b. 40% to 60%
    c. 35% to 55%
    d. 45% to 65%

131. A woman with a healthy pre-pregnancy weight should be advised to gain approximately how much weight during pregnancy?
    a. 25 to 40 pounds
    b. 15 to 25 pounds
    c. 30 to 45 pounds
    d. 25 to 35 pounds

132. Human breast milk contains approximately how many calories per ounce?
    a. 20 calories
    b. 25 calories
    c. 19 calories
    d. 21 calories

133. What is the current recommended folate intake during pregnancy to help reduce the risk of neural tube effects?
    a. 650 mcg
    b. 600 mcg
    c. 750 mcg
    d. 700 mcg

134. By 2030, it is projected that what percentage of adults will be over the age of sixty-five?
   a. One in five
   b. One in six
   c. One in seven
   d. One in eight

135. Aging brings about what changes in body composition?
   a. Fat mass remains the same, visceral fat increases, muscle mass decreases
   b. Fat mass and visceral fat remain the same, muscle mass decreases
   c. Fat mass increases, visceral fat remains the same, muscle mass decreases
   d. Fat mass and visceral fat increase while lean muscle mass decreases

136. Older adults may experience constipation more frequently due to which of the following?
   a. Decreased oral intake
   b. Decreased gastric motility
   c. Decreased fluid intake
   d. All of the above

137. Energy needs annually decline by what percentage?
   a. 3%
   b. 4%
   c. 4.5%
   d. 5%

138. How many minutes of moderate intensity activity is encouraged most days of the week to reduce the risk of chronic disease?
   a. 20 minutes
   b. 30 minutes
   c. 35 minutes
   d. 40 minutes

139. The herbal supplement gingko biloba can interfere with the medication Warfarin because of which of the following reasons?
   a. Decreases how quickly Warfarin is absorbed
   b. Increases how quickly Warfarin is absorbed
   c. Changes blood clotting time
   d. Increases blood clotting

140. What factors must be considered when planning a menu?
   a. Federal regulations
   b. Employee skill level
   c. Operational space
   d. All of the above

Answer Explanations

1. D: Height and weight history is an appropriate part of a physical assessment. Food preferences should be included in the part of the note that includes more subjective information about the patient.

2. D: It is important to evaluate a patient as a whole before making diet recommendations. Medical therapies, life stressors, disease states, underlying conditions, and psychosocial factors all influence an individual's oral intake and ability to digest and absorb nutrients.

3. A: The goal of the Nutritional Assessment of Populations is to gain an understanding of the biological, cultural, and environmental factors that contribute or take away from the nutritional status of communities determined to be at risk. The program also seeks to assess how well-existing programs are serving the health needs of the community and how problem areas identified in the assessment process can be addressed so that health is enhanced.

4. D: Native Americans and Alaskan natives are not eating traditional foods such as deer meat and buffalo as often in favor of food high in calories and saturated fat like hamburgers and fast food. These populations have seen a spike in obesity and obesity-related diseases, such as diabetes.

5. B: A food frequency questionnaire can be administered during a patient appointment to help obtain a diet history. A three-day food record is usually more accurate if food intake is recorded as it is consumed. A twenty-four-hour recall is a quick assessment that can be used to determine what the patient consumed during the previous twenty-four-hour period.

6. A: The Pediatric Nutrition Surveillance System (PedNSS) uses data from the Women, Infants, and Children program (WIC), the Early and Periodic Screening, Diagnosis, and Treatment (EPSDT) Program, and the Title V Maternal and Child Health Program. Data is analyzed to discover trends in birth weight, anemia, breastfeeding, stature, and other nutrition-related indicators. The goal of the program is to use this surveillance data to implement and evaluate existing health programs and formulate public policy.

7. C: If not properly treated and managed, diabetes can lead to many long-term health issues, including blindness, heart disease, stroke, foot and leg problems, and others.

8. A: In diabetes, insulin production is not sufficient or is nonexistent. Therefore, the cells are not able to uptake the glucose that circulates in the blood stream after a meal consumed.

9. D: Keeping carbohydrate intake consistent as much as possible during the day is advice typically given to patients managing Type 2 diabetes. This can help regulate blood sugar levels and prevent spikes in blood sugar during the day.

10. A: A woman who is 5'6" tall with a weight of 130 pounds has a BMI in the healthy range. The formula for calculating BMI is weight (kg)/[height (m)]^2.

11. B: Individuals on insulin therapy should have a regular meal schedule to maximize blood sugar control and prevent a spike or drop in their blood sugar levels. Irregular blood sugar levels can lead to long-term complications.

12. B: The ileum is the part of the small intestine that is most likely involved in Crohn's disease.

13. C: A child with AIDS should consume a diet that is high in calories and high in protein. The increased caloric intake should come from a variety of sources and should not only come from sources of sugar or fat.

14. A: A history of gestational diabetes and a pre-pregnancy BMI greater than thirty places a woman at greater risk for developing gestational diabetes in subsequent pregnancies.

15. D: A baby born to a mother with gestational diabetes is at an increased risk for hypoglycemia at birth and fetal macrosomia, which can cause complications during birth.

16. A: HDL levels should be above 40. Heart disease is a common complication of diabetes, so maintaining higher levels of HDL can provide protective benefits.

17. A: Symptoms of renal insufficiency include anorexia, weakness, weight loss, and vomiting.

18. B: A patient on hemodialysis should aim to maintain a potassium intake of 2 to 3 grams daily. It can also be calculated at 40 mg/kg of ideal body weight.

19. C: People who must avoid milk and all dairy products due to food allergy often struggle with deficiencies in calcium and vitamin D. It is prudent to recommend a safe multivitamin/mineral supplement for individuals avoiding milk and all dairy.

20. C: Because Crohn's disease affects the ileum, certain vitamins and minerals may not be fully absorbed. Individuals with Crohn's disease may require supplements of vitamin C and vitamin B12.

21. B: Whey and casein are the two proteins found in milk. Individuals that need to avoid milk and all dairy products due to a food allergy should avoid any products that contain whey protein.

22. C: Bread made with potato starch is appropriate for someone with Celiac disease. It is important to encourage label reading each time a packaged food is purchased, as ingredients and manufacturing processes can change without warning. A change in the manufacturing process could introduce cross contact with wheat, which would make an item unsafe to eat.

23. A: Vitamin C has been shown in some research studies to be an effective antioxidant and provides cells with protective benefits from free radical damage.

24. C: Individuals undergoing chemotherapy are at greater risk for illness due to a weakened immune system. They should avoid eating raw, undercooked, or unpasteurized foods due to an increased risk of food borne illness.

25. A: The ideal cholesterol intake for persons with heart disease is less than 300 mg per day.

26. B: The DASH (Dietary Approaches to Stop Hypertension) Diet is a Mediterranean-type eating pattern that has been well studied. It has been demonstrated that individuals consuming this type of diet have better controlled blood pressure, which is important in the management and prevention of heart disease.

27. C: Black beans are a good source of folic acid. Organic products are not always fortified, so they may not be a good option for a woman who would like to consume more foods that are high in folic acid.

28. B: In patients with Alzheimer's disease it is important to avoid weight loss and dehydration. Meals should be offered in a quiet, relaxed environment free from distractions such as loud noises and TV.

Meals and snacks should be provided on a regular schedule and self-feeding should be encouraged. Finger foods may help the self-feeding process.

29. D: Symptoms of dehydration include dry mouth, tongue, and mucous membranes; decreased urination; sunken eyes, cheeks, or abdomen; confusion; light-headedness; dizziness; disorientation; dry skin; fatigue; irritability; thirst; and weight loss.

30. B: Foods high in iron include liver, kidney, beef, dried fruits, dried peas and beans, nuts, green leafy vegetables, and fortified whole grain products.

31. C: Pressure ulcers occur when the skin breaks down due to consistent pressure on the same spot and can be found on individuals with limited mobility, poor circulation, have an underlying condition such as diabetes, or can be a warning sign of malnourishment.

32. D: Patients with a diagnosis of anorexia nervosa most likely have many micronutrient deficiencies. It is important to get biochemical labs drawn as quickly as possible and correct electrolyte imbalances prior to feeding the patient to reduce the risk of re-feeding syndrome.

33. B: Individuals suffering with bulimia are often close to a normal weight but may have advanced tooth decay, throat inflammation, damage to their esophagus, and rectal bleeding.

34. B: Avoid excess caffeine and alcohol intake, as these may damage stomach mucosa, making it more difficult for the ulcer to heal and respond to medical therapy.

35. C: Dumping syndrome occurs when large amounts of partially digest food pass into the jejunum. As the body breaks down the food for absorption, large amounts of water are drawn into the intestine in an attempt for the body to achieve osmotic balance.

36. A: Individuals post gastrectomy are at an increased risk for dumping syndrome, as this allows for greater amounts of food to pass to the jejunum. It is often secondary to carbohydrate overload.

37. A: A high fiber diet increases the movement of waste through the colon and decreases intracolonic pressure, relieving symptoms. It can also help reduce the risk of recurring fares.

38. B: Low fiber diets are commonly recommended for individuals managing diverticulitis. Diverticulitis occurs when the diverticula become inflamed as a result of the accumulation of food and residue. As the flare subsides, the patient can gradually return to a high fiber diet.

39. B: While dietary intake plays a role in the development of anemia, individuals with Crohn's disease often experience iron deficiency anemia due to blood loss and decreased absorption.

40. C: During an acute flare of Crohn's disease in which an individual is experiencing diarrhea, it is important to maintain fluid and electrolyte balance. Bowel rest may be needed in cases of severe flares when first line medical therapy that includes an anti-diarrheal agent is not successful.

41. A: Corticosteroids such as prednisone can decrease calcium absorption and can impact bone health in all stages of the life span. This can create a need for an increased amount of calcium and for vitamin D to help protect bone health.

42. B: Steatorrhea is the presence of fat in the stool and is a sign of malabsorption. Treatment should be focused on the underlying condition that is causing the malabsorption.

43. B: Short bowel syndrome occurs when significant sections of the small intestine have been removed and resected. Consequences include malabsorption, malnutrition, fluid and electrolyte imbalances, and weight loss.

44. C: Depending on how much and what sections of the intestine has been lost, supplementation may be needed to accommodate for the loss of absorptive area. Vitamin B12, calcium, iron, and zinc are often needed.

45. A: Total Parental Nutrition (TPN) or nutrition delivered directly into the circulatory system is best following bowel resection surgery to provide gut rest and adequate time to heal. If adequate nutrition is provided, the small intestine will begin to adapt and gradually increase its absorptive capacity.

46. D: Liver failure is defined as the function of the liver being reduced to 30% or less.

47. B: Linoleic acid supplementation is necessary in a diet high in medium chain triglycerides to avoid a deficiency in essential fatty acids.

48. C: Alcohol metabolism requires the use of B vitamins.

49. B: In cirrhosis, damaged liver tissue is replaced by bands of nonfunctional connective tissue that divides the liver into sections and disrupts blood flow.

50. D: The gallbladder stores and concentrates bile. Bile helps in the absorption of fats, vitamins A, D, E, and K, as well as calcium and iron.

51. B: Cholecystitis is inflammation of the gallbladder that causes excess water to be absorbed, allowing cholesterol to precipitate out, which leads to cholelithiasis (gallstones).

52. C: Severe abdominal pain is a symptom of acute pancreatitis. Weight loss, malabsorption, and steatorrhea can develop in cases of chronic pancreatitis.

53. A: An individual with cystic fibrosis requires approximately 120% to 150% of the RDA. The diet should consist of high protein, high calorie, unrestricted fat, and should be liberal in salt.

54. C: In heart failure, the heart muscle is weakened and is unable to pump efficiently, which diminishes blood flow and causes fluid to be held in the tissues. This can lead to edema.

55. A: Excessive levels of uric acid build up in the joints, causing pain and swelling in an individual with gout. This is caused by abnormal metabolism of foods that are high in purine. Examples of high purine foods include broth, anchovies, sardines, organ meats, and sweetbreads.

56. B: An individual develops an endemic goiter from consuming a diet that is low in iodine. This is not common in the United States due to the fortification of table salt, and it is found in common food sources such as seafood, eggs, and milk.

57. C: Anticonvulsants interfere with calcium absorption. Vitamin D supplementation is also required to help reduce the risk of osteomalacia and rickets.

58. D: Anaphylaxis is a severe allergic reaction to a medication or food. It typically involves more than one organ system and can produce systems such as rash, itching, swelling, vomiting, and difficulty breathing. It is life threatening and should be considered a medical emergency.

59. C: Sesame is not considered to be one of the top allergenic foods. The top eight most allergenic foods are milk, wheat, soy, fish, shellfish, peanuts, tree nuts, and eggs.

60. A: Fluid and electrolyte losses from burn wounds can be severe, and the initial treatment period should focus on replacing fluid and electrolytes and maintaining balance.

61. B: Aspirin can decrease the uptake of ascorbic acid and alter the distribution of ascorbic acid in the body, leading to decreased amounts in the body and increased excretion in the urine.

62. A: Corticosteroids can increase protein breakdown, decrease calcium absorption, and decrease protein synthesis. The result can be decreased bone formation, increased excretion of potassium and nitrogen, and increased need for vitamin D.

63. C: Diarrhea is an abnormality of excretion that occurs when stools are frequent and high in liquid content. It is also characterized by an excessive loss of electrolytes, especially sodium and potassium, which can lead to dangerous complications in children.

64. A: Individuals recovering from surgery generally delay oral feeding for 24 to 48 hours, to wait for normal peristalsis to return.

65. D: Patients who do not receive adequate nutrition support in the early post-injury acute stage are at an increased risk of poor wound healing, impaired immune function, and albumin depletion. The severity of the trauma and the resultant injuries determine the amount of carbohydrate and protein needed. Enteral nutrition is routinely given to avoid complications of post-trauma protein loss, which include hypoalbuminemia, infection, slow wound healing, skin breakdown, and reduced immune function, and to meet the nutrition needs for proper healing from a severe injury.

66. B: A BMI under 19 is considered to be underweight, while a BMI in the range of 19 to 24.9 is considered to be a healthy weight. A BMI of 25 to 29.9 classifies one as overweight. A BMI of 30 or greater classifies an individual as obese.

67. A: A diet that provides 500 kcal/day less than required for maintenance should provide weight loss of ~1 lb. a week.

68. C: Chemotherapy is a systemic treatment, and side effects vary according to the drugs and dosage used. Chemotherapy kills rapidly dividing cells, so the entire GI tract may be affected, leading to nausea, vomiting, diarrhea, mouth sores, and inflammation of the esophagus.

69. B: The frequency of consumption of cariogenic food affects caries formation. Eating a large portion of dessert is less damaging than snacking throughout the day.

70. C: Protein malnutrition is common in AIDS patients and can further increase their susceptibility to infections. However, protein intake may be restricted for those with renal disease. Goals of nutritional care include preservation of protein stores, prevention of vitamin or mineral deficiencies that reduce immune status, and treatment of complications that compromise nutritional status.

71. D: AIDS is caused by the blood-borne virus HIV, which destroys T lymphocyte function and therefore causes severe immune deficiency. The virus is also transmitted through breast milk, so HIV positive mothers should not nurse.

72. A: The malnourished state common to COPD patients is thought to be a result of increased energy needs, anorexia, and increased oxygen consumption. The goals of nutritional support include maintaining ideal body weight, managing medication side effects, and managing the edema of patients with cor pulmonale.

73. A: In nutrition diagnostic labeling, functional balance is described as problems that can be physical or mechanical and interfere with one's ability to achieve normal nutrition status. An example is one's ability to swallow properly.

74. B: In nutrition diagnostic labeling, biochemical balance represents a loss of the ability to normally metabolize foods due to medication intake, surgery, or a disease process. An example is the inability to eat wheat due to the diagnosis of Celiac disease.

75. C: In nutrition diagnostic labeling, weight balance describes the involuntary weight changes that can cause a patient to deviate from the patient's normal or desired body weight. An example is rapid, sudden weight loss.

76. B: The intake domain of nutrition diagnosis includes problems related to the ingestion of energy, vitamins, minerals, and fluids, and whether the patient receives nutrition orally, enterally, or parenterally.

77. A: The intake domain in nutrition diagnostic labeling contains the following five classes of concern: calorie energy balance, oral or nutrition support intake, fluid intake balance, bioactive substance charting, and nutrient balance.

78. D: The behavioral-environmental domain describes problems or findings that relate to a patient's knowledge, attitudes, beliefs, environment, food safety, or access to food. Knowledge and beliefs may encompass cultural practices that are harmful to one's nutritional status.

79. C: The PES statement should describe a patient's problem, etiology, signs, and symptoms. It should include the phrases "related to" and "as evidenced by" to be considered complete and easily identifiable in the patient's medical record. The nutrition care plan should clearly outline how nutritional therapy will help return the patient to baseline.

80. A: A therapeutic diet is one that is specifically designed to meet a patient's needs. Therapeutic diets vary widely and can be based on well-studied or popular eating patterns to help the patient find resources after discharge.

81. D: A high calorie, high protein diet is most often ordered for patients who have suffered a high degree of weight loss in a short period of time, those who were not able to eat anything by mouth over an extended period of time, and/or in failure to thrive cases.

82. C: A lacto-vegetarian eats a plant-based diet but also chooses to include milk and dairy items in their diet. Eggs would not be a part of this person's normal eating pattern.

83. B: The ketogenic diet gets its name because the high fat content of the diet results in conversion of fat-to-ketones that are utilized as an energy source in place of glucose. This diet has been shown to be effective in helping patients manage seizure disorders.

84. C: The hemodialysis diet will restrict foods that contain high amounts of sodium, phosphorus, and potassium.

85. B: Reducing sodium intake to less than 1500 mg/day or less can help individuals who are truly salt sensitive; in others it may help the medications work more effectively.

86. A: Nutritional management of galactosemia includes lifelong galactose elimination from the diet. This includes avoiding all dairy products, dates, bell peppers, organ meats, and papaya.

87. D: Formula should be discarded every 24 hours to avoid diarrhea from bacterial contamination.

88. D: A patient with dysphagia to thin liquids is an appropriate candidate for enteral nutrition if they are not willing to drink thickened liquids, placing them at risk for dehydration. Enteral nutrition should be initiated in patients who are not expected to consume an oral diet that will meet their needs within three to five days.

89. B: Refeeding syndrome occurs when aggressive refeeding in a patient who has been without proper food for a period of time causes phosphorus to rapidly leave the plasma and enters the cells in order to become a part of adenosine triphosphate.

90. A: Anyone who has gone for a period of time without proper nutrition can be at risk for refeeding syndrome if refeeding is too aggressive. Alcoholics that typically fast while on drinking binges are at risk for a number of micronutrient deficiencies, which puts them at a greater risk for developing refeeding syndrome.

91. A: The Adult Treatment Panel III reports that individuals with elevated blood pressure, diabetes, family history of heart disease, or who smoke are at an increased risk for heart disease if they have a LDL level over 100.

92. C: The therapeutic lifestyle diet (TLC) recommended by the Adult Treatment Panel III report calls for increased fiber intake (10 to 25 g/day), lowered saturated fat intake (less than 7% calories), and lowered cholesterol intake (less than 200 mg/day). Moderate physical activity and maintaining normal body weight are also recommended.

93. C: The Nutrition Care Process (NCP) was developed to give dietitians a common structure and method to promote better decision-making and to obtain data that may be evaluated quantitatively and qualitatively.

94. D: USDA programs include Commodity Food Donation/Distribution Program, National School Lunch Program, Child and Adult Care Food Program, WIC program, Healthy Start and Head Start, and the Food Stamp Program.

95. B: Nutrition evaluation is a tool used to measure the efficacy of the nutrition intervention on a patient. The evaluation process measures objective outcomes that show that the patient's behavior or health has improved as a result of the service or intervention.

96. C: HIPAA guidelines state that protected health information includes any information that can be used to uniquely identify a patient.

97. A: Myoglobin contributes to the color in beef and changes as the beef is exposed to oxygen. As it oxidizes it changes from red, to brown, to green. A greenish tint in beef indicates extensive breakdown of myoglobin.

98. D: Eggs contribute quite a bit to baked goods. A whole egg added to a baked good contributes vitamins and minerals from the yolk and protein from the white. The color of the yolk also contributes to the final color of a baked good. It helps promote structure by promoting firmness and stability. Beating eggs during the mixing process incorporates air and this retained air contributes to the volume of the baked item.

99. D: Eggs are considered a high quality protein and are the protein by which all other proteins are judged, to determine quality and value to the human body. The albumin (white) contains all of the amino acids that are essential to the human body.

100. A: Ultra High Temperature (UHT) pasteurization sterilizes milk by heating it above the boiling point. Milk that has undergone ultra-high temperature pasteurization can be stored in an airtight container at room temperature for up to six months. This type of pasteurization can alter the flavor of milk. This type of pasteurization does not alter the nutrient value of milk.

101. C: Evaporated milk has had 60% of the water removed. In the United States, it must not contain less than 7.9% milk fat. It usually has a slightly brownish color that is caused by the caramelization of lactose during the canning process.

102. A: Low lactose milk is treated with the enzyme lactase to breakdown lactose. This treatment makes the milk better tolerated by individuals with the condition lactose intolerance. The lactase is added during processing. It is possible for an individual to make their own low lactose milk by adding lactase to regular milk and holding it in the refrigerator.

103. B: Ethylene gas is given off naturally by fruits during the ripening process. Apples are known for giving off the greatest amount of ethylene gas and can cause rapid over ripening if stored with other fruits. The speed at which fruit ripens and the production of ethylene gas can be slowed down by storing fruits in the refrigerator.

104. C: Carotenoids are least affected by the pH of a cooking solution. They are insoluble in water.

105. A: Lycopene contributes the red color in tomatoes and watermelon. It acts as an antioxidant and helps protect cells from damage. Heating a food, such as tomatoes, makes the lycopene more accessible by the body.

106. A: Pectin found in ripe fruit is converted to pectic acid and contributes to the properties of overripe fruit. Pears, apples, citrus fruits, and plums contain large amounts of pectin. Pectin is a soluble fiber.

107. D: Cake flour contains the least amount of protein at 7.5%, pastry flour contains 7.9% protein, and all-purpose flour contains 10% protein, while bread flour contains the most protein at 11.8%. The protein content of flour contributes to the structure of baked goods.

108. C: Gluten does not contribute any color to a baked product. It does contribute to the elastic properties of baked goods, forms the framework, and helps hold in leavening agents.

109. B: Adding fat to a baked good contributes to the tenderness of the product. It achieves this by coating the gluten particles and prevents the gluten from over-developing, which can contribute to a tough baked good.

110. A: Engineered foods are made by inserting the genes from one organism into another organism. This can be accomplished by transferring the genes from plants, animals, bacteria or other microorganisms into another plant or animal. This continues to be a controversial practice, with proponents stating this creates plants that grow faster, are more drought tolerant, and pest resistant. Opponents state that the modified organisms can crossbreed with natural organisms and cause environmental harm.

111. B: Yogurt can be considered a functional food. Functional foods are foods that have a positive influence on human health beyond basic nutrition. Functional foods can be naturally occurring or can be made through fortification. Yogurt that has been cultured with beneficial bacteria contributes to overall gut health in addition to providing other nutrients such as protein and calcium.

112. C: Dry heat cooking methods are best suited for cuts of meat with less connective tissue. Connective tissue can be difficult to break down. If not fully broken down during the cooking process, the final product will be tough and dry.

113. D: Moist heat cooking methods require the use of water or another cooking liquid. Examples of moist heat cooking methods include braising, simmering, steaming, and stewing.

114. C: Nitrates and Nitrites are food additives added to processed meats to inhibit the growth of C. botulinum spores. Other food additives are used to fix color, prevent browning, are emulsifiers, and are stabilizers.

115. A: Carbohydrates contribute 4 kilocalories per gram.

116. A: Protein contributes 4 kilocalories per gram.

117: D: Fat contributes 9 kilocalories per gram.

118: C: Starch is one of the most abundant sources of carbohydrates in the typical diet.

119. A: Omega-3 fatty acids are important polyunsaturated fat and must come from food sources. Good sources of these fatty acids include fish, ground flax seeds, walnuts, canola oil, and soybean oil.

120. D: Micronutrients are vitamins and minerals and are only needed in small quantities. They must be obtained from the diet to support a healthy immune system, tissue repair, growth and development in children, and overall health and wellbeing. Iodine and zinc are micronutrients. Macronutrients, in contrast, are needed in large quantities.

121. D: National Nutrient Database for Standard Reference contains nutrient information on almost 9,000 foods and is maintained by the Nutrient Data Laboratory. Special interest databases include Flavonoids, Isoflavones, and Proanthocyanidins.

122. C: Macronutrients are carbohydrates, fats, and protein that are important sources of energy for the body and are needed in large quantities. They contribute to the overall energy pool of the body.

123. C: Glucose is the only substrate utilized by the brain.

124. A: Digestion begins in the mouth during the process of chewing food and continues in the stomach and concludes in the small intestine. Digestion is an important physiological process breaking down macro- and micro- nutrients into smaller, more easily absorbed forms that can be utilized by the body.

125. B: Insulin is an important hormone that regulates blood sugar levels. Cholecystokinin (CCK) is secreted by the proximal small bowel and stimulates the pancreas to secrete enzymes, slows gastric emptying, stimulates gallbladder contraction and colonic activity, and may regulate appetite. Secretin is released from the duodenal wall and stimulates the pancreas to secrete water and bicarbonate. It inhibits gastric acid secretion and stomach emptying. Secretin is stimulated by the presence of food in the stomach and the smell or sight of food. Wine, caffeine, food extracts, or partially digested proteins can stimulate secretin production and release. Gastrin is produced in the stomach and stimulates gastric secretions and motility.

126. B: The metabolic rate in the human body is affected by several variables including body size and composition, age, gender, and hormonal status. External factors such as the intake of caffeine, nicotine, and alcohol use also influences metabolic rate.

127. C: Excretion is necessary for the human body to eliminate waste products from metabolism. The major organs involved in excretion are the skin, lungs, kidneys, liver, large intestine, and gall bladder.

128. C: Of all life stages, infants require the most calories, fat, protein, and water per gram of body weight. Between birth and six months, a normally developing infant requires approximately 550 calories per day, 9.1 grams of protein, and a minimum of 30 grams of fat per day. Fluid needs are based on age and range between 125 and 155 mL per kilogram of body weight. Between six and twelve months, normally developing infants require approximately 700 calories per day, 13.5 grams of protein, and still require a minimum of 30 grams of fat daily. Fluid needs can be calculated at 1.5 mL per calorie or based on body weight.

129. B: A normally developing child experiences the most rapid rate of growth during infancy and adolescence.

130. D: For a healthy adult, carbohydrates should make up approximately 45% to 65% of total calories, fat should make up approximately 20% to 35% of total calories, while protein should make up the balance; approximately 10% to 35%

131. D: A healthy woman with no other diseases or underlying conditions who was at a healthy weight prior to pregnancy should be advised to gain between 25 and 35 pounds during pregnancy to meet the demands of the fetus and help her return to her healthy pre-pregnancy weight.

132. A: Human breast milk contains approximately 20 calories per ounce. Infant formulas also contain approximately 20 calories per ounce.

133. B: Pregnant women should get about 600 mcg of folate daily to reduce risk of neural tube defects.

134. A: One in five adults will be over the age of sixty-five by 2030, so this is a rapidly growing segment of the American population.

135. D: Aging brings about body composition changes. Fat mass and visceral fat increase while lean muscle mass decreases. This can impact a person's ability to safely engage in physical activity.

136. D: Decreased dietary intake and fluid intake contribute to the development of constipation. However, older adults may experience increased cases of constipation with normal oral intake due to decreased gastric motility.

137. A: Energy needs decline by approximately 3 percent per decade due to sarcopenia and natural decreases in physical activity.

138. B: Current recommendations state 30 minutes of moderate intensity activity is encouraged most days of the week to reduce the risk of chronic disease.

139. C: Gingko biloba changes blood clotting time and can interfere with Warfarin, which is a medication prescribed to individuals with blood clotting disorders.

140. D: Planning a menu is a multifaceted task that must be well thought out over a period of time. First, federal regulations may be in place regarding menu item names and nutrient content of foods. Secondly, the skill level of the employees will dictate the type of menu items abled to be executed properly. Employees with little to no food service experience will not likely be able to achieve a five-course meal in a nice restaurant. The operational space must also be considered when planning a menu. A kitchen only accommodating two cooks/chefs should not have a menu with countless options.

Food Science and Food Service

Menu Development

Mealtimes are often the bright spot in someone's day. Food should not only be tasty, but also be attractive to the eye, nutritionally sound, and safe to eat. Creating menus that satisfy these four standards embodies numerous considerations. Other aspects to consider include federal regulations, cultural beliefs and practices, clinical diet of consumer, skill set of staff, budget, and production space.

Types of Menus

Nonselective, Selective Menus
A menu is a list of food items offered in an establishment that may be ordered or served. The information displayed in a menu varies based on the institution for which the institution is used. A selective menu includes two or more food choices in each menu category available. Categories include appetizers, salads, vegetables/side dishes, entrees, and desserts. On the contrary, a nonselective menu only offers one food choice or one menu category.

Cycle, Static Menus
Menus can be static or cyclic. A static menu is often found in restaurants where the same menu is used daily, in part because the consumer is changing daily. Having a variety of consumers each day allows for a static menu to seem non-repetitive. Generally, static menus are also selective menus, which contain numerous choices. Benefits to a static menu include consistency, production ease, simpler waste control, and higher customer appreciation. Static menus can have disadvantages as well. These menus are often labor intensive, include out-of-season items or ingredients, and have too many choices. Cyclic menus are a series of menus that are rotated and repeated at fixed time intervals. These time intervals vary upon the establishment, but may be weekly, monthly, bimonthly, etc. Both selective and nonselective menus can be used in a cycle. Advantages include reduced time spent menu planning, increased efficiency of production, and increased standardization of recipes and production. Disadvantages of cyclic menus may involve repetitiveness when the cycle is too short, especially in a long-term care setting. Deciding between a static or cycle menu is dependent on the frequency of the clientele and establishment type, as well as the number of menu items available.

Retail, Restaurant, Room Service
Food service establishments are numerous. The three most common are retail, restaurant, and room service. Retail food includes all food that is purchased by a consumer and consumed off-premise, excluding restaurant food. Grocery stores, convenient stores, mass merchandisers, and drug stores all sell retail food. Retail food can also be purchased from health foods stores, online, or by mail order, and it may be perishable or non-perishable. Retail food outlets must determine what foods customers will purchase and in what quantities, what the building and supplies can accommodate, and where to source their products. Of the three categories, retail food is consumed the most compared to restaurant or room service.

Restaurant menus can be static or cyclic and can be selective or non-selective, or a combination of such variables. Due to different foods being available during different seasons, restaurants may opt for cyclic menus that change each season. Larger franchise restaurants often have a static, selective menu in order to establish consistency despite numerous owners and managers. Small-scale restaurants may find it better suited for their clientele to have selective menus that change more frequently.

Room service menus are typically used in hotel establishments as well as acute and long-term care facilities. Menus are generally selective and static. Room service menus typically feature both prepared meal items and a la carte items. In acute and long-term care facilities, various room service menus may be available based on the clinical diet prescribed by a Registered Dietitian. Typically, patients or customers are able to order from the room service menus whenever they need to. This creates less food waste due to the consumer only ordering when hungry. Menu items are made to order, allowing for fresher meals served to the consumer.

Menu Development

Guidelines

Federal regulations authorize that institutions must provide each consumer with a meal that is nutritious, edible, tasty, and incorporates a balance of macro and micronutrients suitable to the dietary requirements and any special dietary needs present. A menu must be created in advance and adhered to. All food must be prepared per standardized recipes and prepared and served to correct temperatures to avoid food-borne illnesses. If a patient has certain nutritive practices or a prescribed clinical diet, menu modifications and substitutions must be available and deliver comparable nutritional values. Federal regulations mandate that facilities must have at least three scheduled mealtimes each day relative to common times for breakfast, lunch, and dinner, with no more than fourteen hours between dinner and breakfast; however, if a snack is provided after dinner, sixteen hours may elapse between dinner and breakfast.

In the event that a consumer needs assistive devices at meal times, the care facility must provide them. Assistive devices include but are not limited to:

- Lip plate
- Cup
- Weighted utensils
- Feeding devices
- Paid feeding assistant

Paid feeding assistants should be trained and work under the supervision of a licensed or registered nurse. Training must be conducted through a state-approved course, which contains at least eight hours and includes feeding techniques, communication and social skills, proper responses to resident behavior, assistance with hydration and feeding, safety and emergency techniques (ex. Heimlich maneuver), infection control, respecting resident rights, and acknowledging and documenting change in behavior. The paid feeding assistants are not trained or permitted to feed patients who have difficulty swallowing, experience aspiration of the lungs, or utilize a feeding tube.

Clients

Profiling clients is necessary to determine what they want to see on a menu and order. Establishing a goal for the atmosphere and reputation of an institution is important in determining what customers expect with ordering and consuming when purchasing food from the menu.

Operational Influences

When planning a menu, not only do federal regulations need to be considered, but also the potential and capability of the operation and operational space. The operation's overall goal or concept will also dictate decisions. When considering recipes for a menu, it is crucial to ensure that the equipment and staff available are able to execute the expectations. For example, it is not likely that a meal can be successfully cooked and held to proper temperatures while maintaining the integrity of the foods' profiles if all menu items must be prepared using one piece of equipment. Creating a menu that utilizes multiple areas of the kitchen is necessary to ensure food is prepared as close to service time as possible. If certain staff members are limited in their capabilities, it is not wise to have many food items with extensive preparation needs at one meal. If an operation wishes to serve as a fast-casual dining concept, it must serve first-class items in a fraction of the time and at a fraction of the cost as an up-scale restaurant. Equipment and staff available must allow for the promise of quality food made quickly. The budget of the operation is a strong dictator in food items that can be incorporated in a menu. Typically, a mix of higher and lower priced food items make for a well-balanced menu choice for two reasons. First, customers will see value in the entrée with the higher priced food item. Second, the food service institution will still be able to make a profit on the entrée, due to the pairing with lower priced food. Avoiding or restricting the incorporation of foods whose price fluctuates greatly can limit a negative impact financially.

External Influences/Contingencies
Focusing on the operational influences in an institution is important in directing the menu development; however, external factors exist that play a role in developing the menu. Competition is one external factor. Not only is price a factor in competition, but also food quality, taste, presentation, atmosphere, and location. Competitors should be identified for restaurants to differentiate from in order to attract customers. Competition also exists among food and product distributers. Shopping the market to determine which company offers foods that meet the operation's standards at a reasonable cost, while delivering at times and frequencies suitable to the operation, is crucial. Establishing a relationship with the distributor decreases the risk of deliveries being late, incorrect, or mishandled. Another external factor is the pricing of food; food prices fluctuate depending on availability, season, and weather. If applicable, institutions will have to make a decision to change prices or not, based on alterations in food prices.

Contingencies that may affect an operation are renovations, natural disasters, or emergencies (fire, robbery, etc.). Renovations may limit appliances available for cooking, preparation space, and service area. Typically, renovations involve improving areas or methods; however, the renovation process may hinder the ability to create certain menu items. The capability to store food properly may also be altered during times of renovation. Natural disasters are known to affect the food supply around the world. If California experiences a drought, produce items such as nuts and fruit may experience a shortage, causing prices to rise. Though the operation may be hundreds of miles from California, the food distributor used may source produce from California. When food costs go up, unchanged menu prices result in smaller profit margins and, in some cases, a loss. Emergencies such as a fire in the kitchen may damage equipment necessary to prepare menu items. Due to the large costs of commercial kitchen equipment, it may be difficult for an establishment to replace it immediately.

Client/Customer Satisfaction
Customer or client satisfaction is crucial in a successful business. An organization needs to measure satisfaction, to determine if customers' expectations are met. Satisfaction can be evaluated by looking at various factors. The first factor is sales. Looking at sales trends from month to month and year to year will give some insight into the success of the operation's ability to please the customer. A second factor in evaluating satisfaction is client feedback. Many businesses provide an avenue for customers to provide feedback and evaluate their experience. Collecting the data is necessary, but evaluation cannot stop there. Evaluating and analyzing the data collected is required to extract the results to clarify if changes are necessary. Documenting findings in an organized manner makes the data useful and accessible for comparison in future studies. The final step in evaluating customer satisfaction is

implementing change, if necessary. If a common complaint among customers is an unclean eating area, an obvious remedy is mandating that the dining room be cleaned more frequently. More difficult solutions are required for complaints of high menu pricing. The operation must then go back to standardized recipes to determine how to improve the customers' perception of cost-value.

Menu Modifications

Menu modifications can be a result of food sensitivities, clinical needs, allergies, and cultural practices. In acute and long-term care facilities, various clinical diets exist, requiring pureed food, restricted calories or carbohydrates, low sodium foods, vegetarian, or ground up foods. Food preferences and allergies also exist in this setting. As mentioned, federal regulation mandates alternative menu items must be available that are comparable to the original menu item. Restaurants are also faced with customers who have sensitivities, allergies, or nutrition practices. While it is not federally mandated to provide alternative options, satisfying the customer is less likely without alternative choices. Because consumers normally follow trends, restaurants must also decide to follow trends or stick to their menu. For example, the number of people following a gluten-free diet has skyrocketed in the past five years. Many restaurants have followed their customers on this trend and now offer gluten-free menu options for foods that normally contain gluten. While this is a costly practice, businesses may see more of a benefit to offer trendy items to customers.

Procurement and Supply Management

Developing Specifications for Purchase of Food/Supplies

Quality standards must first be determined of the food and other supplies used in a food service establishment. Suppliers offer many products and services that vary greatly in quality. Therefore, the operation must determine the quality standard for each product or food item used, as well as for service. Quality standards identify characteristics and specifications for each product purchased for service. In order to offer a consistent product, it is essential that these standards be communicated to associates in the establishment. The quality standards must also be well documented and include detailed descriptions of the expectations of products and services. Documentation should include:

- Writing record of purchasing criteria so the business preserves control over quality and cost of all purchases

- Identify specific requirements for products or services for current and future bids

- Define a replacement policy, clearly communicated with the distributor in the event that products delivered do not meet specifications

The expected level of quality of the operation must be identified. For example, a five-star restaurant would not purchase very low-grade meat and sell it as high-grade meat. If a fast-casual restaurant determines lower grade meat is appropriate for their clientele, menu style, and location, they would purchase a lower grade meat. The fast-casual restaurant may also decide plastic utensils and paper napkins reduce labor costs and fit the environment; however, a five-star steakhouse would opt for real silverware and linen napkins.

Once quality standards are established, product specifications can be set to meet those standards. Product specifications illustrate the requisite characteristics of a service or product, as well as how a product is purchased. Large chain operations may be limited to approved suppliers for products and services; however, these large scale agreements may offer additional services such as free delivery or preferred shipping and delivery times. The larger businesses may also have more extensive specifications, in order to maintain consistency across locations. On the contrary, smaller independent operations may have more lenient specifications that only list a couple requirements. It is important to inform the distributor of the business's needs, to successfully deliver what is expected. Product specifications generally include the intended use of the product or service, the exact name for an item, the brand of the item, the correct packaging, the size of the product, the acceptable trim measures, the U.S. grade of the item (if applicable), the type of preservation or processing method, the color, the place of origin, acceptable substitutes, unit pricing, pricing limits, and temperature control procedures.

The intended use of the product describes how the item will be used, developed, or consumed. The intended use should drive the decisions for the rest of the specifications. For example, when catering a dinner meal to 300 people, having individual butter packets instead of tubs of butter on the table for rolls may be more cost-effective for that evening. Once an economy-sized butter container is opened, it has limited shelf life; however, the individualized butter packets that go unused can be used again. The quality specification would identify the need for real butter; however, the product specification would detail the need for individual servings of butter, due to its intended use.

The exact name for an item is essential, especially for items with multiple flavors and color variations. Using the correct name will help ensure the exact product desired is received. For example, if ordering mayonnaise, mayonnaise can be made with olive oil, canola oil, or the original recipe. If the clientele is health conscious, it may be necessary to order olive oil mayonnaise instead of regular. Specifying the brand name and product will lower possibilities for error.

Specific brand names should be documented where applicable. People are often influenced to purchase services or products based on the brand name. For this reason, it is important to consider if the product or service will be presented to the consumer in any way. If so, it may be best to specify a brand name item. If not, a generic brand that matches the quality standards indicated may suit the operation better.

Many products come in different packaging options. Products may be packaged in various manners based on storage, transportation, use, and cost. For example, mustard can be purchased in commercial-sized cans, bottles, or small packets. A fast-food or delivery set-up may benefit from individualized small packets of mustard; a casual sit down restaurant may choose to put bottles of mustard on the tables, and a more formal institution may benefit from a bulk packaging to serve mustard in ramekins. Considering which packaging is best also relies on the frequency of use. If a food product is perishable, the type of packaging will play a large role in the integrity of the food once it arrives to the destination.

The required size of the product is included in the specifications. The size includes weight measurements, weight ranges, or counts. Identifying serving sizes required for the specific food product in the standardized recipes plays a key role in understanding how much is used each day/week. In addition, calculating how many of that menu item is sold each service is also necessary when determining needs.

Edible yield is included in defining specifications for food products. Edible yield is the amount of food that is served to the consumer after it has been washed, trimmed, and prepared. Products with higher waste and lower edible yield are cheaper than products with little to no waste.

The United States Department of Agriculture (USDA) grades are used for over 300 different food and agricultural items, with the goal of providing quality measurements or indicators for consumers. Eggs, poultry, beef, and other food items are USDA graded. The grade determines the quality and value of the product. Depending on the type of establishment, different quality of grades may be more appropriate. USDA prime, USDA choice, and USDA select are examples of grades for beef.

The preservation or processing method, also called the market form, indicates how an item is processed before it is packaged. The market form can apply to many food types. For example, chicken breast may be formed into nuggets before packaging for shipment. Another example is strawberries. Strawberries may be fresh, sliced, or frozen. Other items like garlic can be fresh, minced, or dried. The item's use will pinpoint the correct product to order.

When applicable, purchasers must specify what color product is desired. Choosing between red grapes or green grapes is essential to be sure desired products are received. Colors may be important for the flavor profile as well. Green and red grapes offer different tastes, which can alter a recipe. Thus, specifying colors of products are important in executing menu items correctly.

The place of origin of a product indicates exactly where a food item is coming from. This standard is significant due to a number of factors:

- An institution's menu may state that an ingredient is from a certain region
- The flavor and texture of a food may vary from region to region
- Policies may dictate products must not come from a certain region
- Operations may market serving local food to guarantee quality

Due to many circumstances, specified items may not be available. Acceptable substitutes that are selected during the specification process can save time and effort if the primary product is unavailable. Acceptable substitute items come from the same distributor. Substitutes must not alter recipes or appearance. Substitutes should be tested to ensure no alterations are made to menu items and that the product still meets the consumers' expectations as well as the primary item.

Price is a key determinant in choosing food items that are appropriate for the operation's use. Unit pricing is just what it explains; it is the price per unit identified. This measure is important in pinpointing which product is economically wise for the institution to purchase based on its usage. The unit price can help determine if it is better to buy by the pound or case for items.

Because pricing is subject to change, based on the availability and economy, price limits must be set for products and food used in production. The vendor may not ship the product if the cost exceeds the price limit. If the price continues to exceed the maximum, the purchaser must find an acceptable substitute, raise the maximum, or choose to no longer order the product.

Many perishable items are sensitive to temperatures. When creating specifications, temperatures must be considered in order to guarantee that temperature-sensitive products will be transported and delivered at the specified temperatures. Delivering and receiving temperatures of individual food items must be documented with each delivery. This tedious yet crucial task minimizes the risk for food-borne illnesses. Foods that require temperatures are dairy products, meat, fish, produce, and other beverages. Acceptable temperatures vary based on the food product; however, each food product's appropriate receiving temperature should be clearly documented and available for the receiver. Once delivered, it is imperative that the perishable items are stored in the appropriate place quickly to maintain quality and freshness.

<u>Product and Packaging Selection</u>

Defining the specifications for products is essential in a food service operation. The previous section discussed the numerous factors and parts of a specification for a single item including the intended use, the name and brand of an item, the packaging and size of the product, the U.S. Grade, the market form, color, place of origin, substitutes, pricing, and temperature controls. Adhering to these quality standards set by the purchaser helps to create a plan of action for the purchaser and distributer. Adhering to the standards by the distributer and receiver generates positive results. Many factors can affect the quality standards and should be considered when selecting products for the operation.

The intended use of an item is the most prominent factor in selecting product to order. For example, any fruit or herb that is used as a garnish should be presentable and full of color with great shape; however, herbs that are used in a recipe can be somewhat wilted or not in a desired shape.

The concept and goals of an establishment will dictate all determinants regarding budget, the menu, and employees' skill levels. A five-star restaurant whose goal is for the customer to enjoy and experience along with a high-quality meal will have much different standards than a long-term care facility who receives minimal reimbursement for patients' meals; therefore, items and equipment purchased to carry out the concept and goals must coincide. A tray-line system will fit better in a hospital or long-term care facility than a five-star restaurant, due to the goals and concepts identified.

Often times, the menu is the first deliverance of the product to the consumer. The menu must also display the concept and goals in food form. In the example of the five-star restaurant and long-term care facility, a choice of five seafood entrees is more appropriate to the restaurant than the long-term care facility. If a name brand is mentioned on the menu, the operation is required to specify in the quality standards and order that name brand item only.

The employee skill level also plays a factor in quality standards. Hiring highly skilled employees allows for the ability for more complicated dishes and preparation; however, highly skilled means higher pay. Choosing to make or buy a menu item is something to be considered when selecting food products. Factors to be contemplated in this decision are:

- Consistency
- Cost effectiveness
- Time effectiveness
- Space savings

Value-added products offer consistent portion sizes and quality each time. This allows for the operation to preplan par levels more easily, decreasing the waste each service or day. Pre-packaged products also decrease preparation time, which lowers labor cost and frees time for other tasks that need completion. Because little to no prep is needed, prep and equipment space may be minimized when choosing value-added menu items. In some cases, it may be a better option to make a product in-house. Generally, products made in-house require minimal equipment, storage, and preparation space. Quality standards set by the operation may be better suited for items made in-house than those of value-added items. Connecting with the concepts and goals of the operation to determine the skills necessary for successful service is imperative, not only during the hiring process, but also during the selection of food products and equipment.

Quality versus quantity is an ongoing decision when choosing products for the operation. The budget should be a reflection of the overall concept of the establishment. Each material and product will be influenced by the budget, so it is vital to have an established budget before selecting items.

Ultimately, the customers should be one of the largest factors in quality standards because that will be who is buying the product. Quality standards should not be addressed only in the beginning of an operation, but should be a continual measurement throughout service. Customers, trends, and products change. Being proactive in updating quality standards is necessary for a successful business.

Vendor Selection

Selecting a vendor who is reliable, ethical, financially stable, and able to deliver the unique needs of an operation is crucial to success. There are two types of procurement plans that an operation can choose. The first plan involves the purchaser selecting one to two suppliers to fulfill all of the buying needs of the establishment. For small-scale businesses, this plan is implemented. Larger operations may elect to receive bids from various suppliers for goods and services used. The lowest price should not automatically be selected. Institutions must consider the quality of goods and the reliability of services when selecting the winning bids. Bid buying does not always result in large operations buying all products and services from one supplier. They may choose to use one supplier for produce, one supplier for linen washing, and another for non-food items.

Extensive research should be conducted when picking the supplier that best fits the operation. Understanding the suppliers' business models is just as important as forming the operation's business model. The supplier may outsource delivery services to third party vendors, in which case provides another company to be evaluated in terms of integrity and reliability of services. There are many verification points when selecting suitable vendors:

- The USDA must grade egg, meat, and poultry products sourced by suppliers.
- Suppliers' facilities and trucks should be sanitary.
- Local, state, and federal laws applicable to the service of the supplier must be adhered to.
- References should be provided to confirm supplier's reputability.
- Suppliers' delivery trucks must be able to maintain proper temperatures of items ordered.
- Inspected suppliers must have Hazard Analysis and Critical Control Point (HAACP) program in place.
- Suppliers must have personal hygiene practice procedures in place for personnel.

Once a supplier or suppliers are selected, a contract must be put in place to ensure all expectations on both parties are met. This contract should stipulate who can and cannot accept deliveries. To reduce or eliminate confusion, it is best to have a representative of the supplier to the establishment to identify anything that could make the delivery process difficult, review the receiving area, and establish delivery times and days suitable to both parties. Evaluating suppliers should occur annually. Documenting any issues that occur between the operation and supplier is necessary for corrective action to take place. Before renewing the contract, it is important to conduct a thorough review of what exactly the contract states. The operation may discover that certain procedures or requirements did not work previously, and in such cases, possible changes that would best suit the establishment should be discussed.

Policies and Procedures

The procurement process stems from the operation's concept and goals and clarifies product selection. The ordering, receiving, and storing methods as well as the policies and procedures involved are all components of the procurement process.

<u>Purchasing Systems, Methods, and Decisions</u>
The first step in creating the procurement process is to assess the wants and needs of the operation. A goods and services assessment reviews what it has verses what it ideally needs. While this assessment is often completed by the purchaser, input must be received by employees who use the purchased items daily. For example, chefs should provide input regarding the frequency of ordering products. A chef may notice that certain ingredients that are not used multiple times per day are going to waste. A dining room manager may observe seat cushions ripping over time. Product specifications can be figured out once a thorough assessment is completed.

Selecting criteria and quality standards is the second step in the procurement process. The purchaser carries a large responsibility in the standards for an operation's products. There are countless selection factors affecting product selection that include, but are not limited to: intended use, U.S. government grades, type of container, color, degree of ripeness, supplier services, lifetime cost, appearance, ease of cleaning, energy source, warranty, code compliance, and quality.

Once the goods and services needs assessment is conducted and products are selected, defining ordering procedures is next. Ordering procedures vary based on the different suppliers and operations. Phone or form orders are often used. In some establishments, the purchaser is in charge of determining what needs to be ordered. In larger operations, managers of each section are responsible to submit a purchase requisition of what is needed in their respective sections. To keep procedures streamlined, the sequence of events must be established. Managers must place desired orders to purchasers by certain dates, detailing what is needed and by what date. Documentation of such orders should be provided to the respective manager, the vendor, the receiver, and the accountant, if applicable. Documentation ensures that all parties are aware of the order status. A replacement or return policy must be in place in the event that a delivery does not meet the quality standards set by the operation. This should be clearly noted in the contract.

Step four involves defining receiving procedures—a crucial step in assuring what was ordered was actually received. Receiving orders is a tedious process that ensures the operation is adhering to its concept and goals. To alleviate some stress in receiving orders, a suitable receiving dock that is clean, secure, well lit, and well located are practical characteristics for the location. Each operation should have appropriate receiving equipment, which may include calibrated thermometers, scales, pallet jack, and calculators. It is important to assign a responsible and well-trained associate to receive the shipment and check for all items ordered and to follow all receiving procedures. Prior to the contract being signed, the supplier and receiver should designate a day and time that orders will be delivered and received. A copy of the purchase order must be available and on hand when the order arrives. This document is to be compared with the supplier's invoice to ensure the full order is received. Orders received must be checked and accepted or refused with proper documentation.

The final step in the procurement process is having proper storage places for all items. This includes freezer items, refrigerated items, paper goods, cleaning supplies, and shelf-stable items. Larger operations will have a separate employee to put the order away to reduce the risk of theft, whereas smaller institutions may not find it beneficial to increase labor costs for this purpose.

A flowchart should be created to identify the main steps in creating the procurement process:

1. Assess the wants and needs of the operation
2. Select criteria and quality standards for the service and food of the operation
3. Define ordering procedures
4. Create receiving procedures
5. Ensure proper storage room for ordered items

Inventory Management

Managing inventory is essential in the food service business. An inventory control system should be very sound to allow for enough food items to be on hand to serve the demands of the customers, while not having too much that some is wasted. To master this balance, purchasers evaluate product turnover rate, or the amount of time it takes for the inventory to move from the operation's receiving dock to the consumer.

The percentage of sales volume estimate is another consideration in managing inventory. Many theories exist on what the correct percentage is; however, an operation should establish a percentage in the policies and procedures.

Inventory turnover and percentage of sales volume fail to indicate specific product pars and usage. In order to determine the usage of a certain product, the expected usage of food, nonfood, and beverage items must be calculated for the stated period.

Historical usage data is used as a starting point in calculating usage. Historical usage data consists of an item's popularity index, customer count histories, and external factors that may affect sales. The number of customers expected in the upcoming period, or customer count forecast, can be computed with this formula:

$$\text{Customer Count last Period} + \left(\text{customer count last period} \times \text{\% increase expected}\right) = \text{Customer Count forecast this Period}$$

Once this number is obtained, it can be multiplied by the popularity index to forecast the usage. To calculate the popularity index, the number of customers choosing a particular entrée is divided by the total number of entrées sold. Multiplying the popularity index by the customer count forecast for a certain period will determine the forecasted supply of a particular item for the given period. Once the forecasted number is calculated, figuring the amount of the food item to order depends on the operation's use of the Levinson approach or par stock approach.

The Levinson method predicts the amount of product to order based on a specific period's consumed portion size relative to the sales volume of a particular item. In order to predict the amount of product, it is necessary to determine the total amount of each ingredient to order. The portion factor is the number of portions found in the appropriate measurement for an item. For example, if a recipe calls for 4 ounces of pork loin, dividing 1 pound (16 ounces) by the serving size of 4 ounces determines that the portion factor is 4. The portion divider is calculated by multiplying the portion factor by the edible yield percentage of the specified ingredient. If the edible yield of the pork loin is 75 percent, the portion divider is 3. Once the portion factor and portion divider are calculated, the order size can be determined by dividing the item's usage by the ingredient's portion divider. Given the case that 1,789 consumers will eat the 4 ounces pork loin, the operation should order 597 pounds of pork loin. Below are the calculations for each of the steps above.

portion factor (PF) = 1 pound (16 ounces) ÷ amount of an ingredient needed for 1 serving

portion factor (PF): 16oz.÷ 4 oz = 4

portion divider (PD) = portion factor(PF) × ingredients edible yield percentage

portion divider (PD): 4 ÷ 0.75 = 3

Order size = Number of customers who will consume item ÷ ingredient's PD

Order size: 1,789 ÷ 3 = 596.3 lbs or 597 lbs

The par stock approach determines the level of inventory for each specific item needed for production to meet the consumer demand from one delivery date to the next. This method is much simpler than the Levinson method and consists of the following steps:

- Establish the supplier's delivery schedule.

- All inventory items must have a par stock level. Various factors should be included in determining this level. Considerations should comprise of sales projections of menu items. Sales projections must reflect ordering trends due to seasons, product availability, sales and promotions, or other features. Ordering dates will come before the delivery date for an amount of time that is based on the contract between the supplier and the establishment. Deciding par levels in advance for the time between delivery dates is necessary to maintain inventory for production without wasting product. Establishing par stock depends on storage space for nonperishables and figuring the frequency of deliveries for perishables.

- Prior to placing orders, the historical usage data for that time period should be considered. Current trends of menu item sales as well as upcoming events (such as private parties with a special menu, banquet, conference, catering orders, etc.) at the establishment for the ordering period should be analyzed next. The order quantity is then calculated by deducting what is currently in stock from the par stock level. Lastly, additional needs based on the events that ordering period are added.

Par stock levels should be revisited when there are changes in delivery schedules, or when there are changes in popularity of menu items. This approach is popular due to the simplicity of calculating, and the predictability of deliveries. The par stock approach is suitable for fairly static menus. One downfall of this approach is that it does not focus on food costs like the Levinson method.

Both the par stock and Levinson approach are necessary methods in ordering proper quantities of items used in production; however, considering the costs associated with ordering and storing inventory also impacts how much is ordered and at what frequency.

A sample par stock sheet is shown below:

Item Name	Order Unit	Unit Price	Par Level	Day 1 On Hand	Day 1 Order	Day 2 On Hand	Day 2 Order	Day 3 On Hand	Day 3 Order	Day 4 On Hand	Day 4 Order
Bacon, Sliced	lb	2.99	20 lb								
Beef Patty, 8 oz. Angus Chuck	lb	2.49	30 lb								
Beef, Eye Round	lb	2.29	40 lb								
Beef, Inside Angus	lb	2.09	40 lb								
Beef, Ground	lb	2.09	60 lb								
Beef, Liver	lb	3.29	15 lb								
Beef, Ribeye	lb	2.99	60 lb								
Beef, Red Brisket	lb	2.29	40 lb								

Storage costs, or the product's carrying cost, is defined as the summation of all the costs associated with properly storing nonfood items, food items, and beverages from the moment they are received to the moment they are consumed. Included in storage costs are the costs of insurance and maintenance of the storage facility, as well as the costs acquired from spoilage or expired items. The largest component of storage cost is the opportunity cost or capital cost. Opportunity cost exemplifies how much money is invested in the inventory and therefore is not able to be used for any other purpose. The purchaser must consider both the storage and ordering costs when calculating the correct order size and time. The most effective amount to order is termed the economic order quantity (EOQ) and can be calculated in dollars and in number of units. Below are equations to determine each method:

$$\sqrt{\frac{2 \times \text{ordering cost per order (in dollars)} \times \text{amount of item used in one year (in dollars)}}{\text{storage costs per year as a percentage of average dollar value of inventory}}}$$
$$= \text{EOQ in dollars}$$

$$\sqrt{\frac{2 \times \text{ordering cost per order (in dollars)} \times \text{amount of item used in one year (in units)}}{\text{storage costs per year as a percentage of average dollar value of inventory}}}$$
$$= \text{EOQ in units}$$

If an establishment calculates the number of pounds of pork loin based on consumer demand and figures 597 pounds are necessary for the upcoming period, using the EOQ equations will help determine the correct amount to order. Historical usage data shows the operation uses 10,542 pounds of pork loin annually. The cost of one pound is $2.25; however, the contract between the operation and supplier notes the supplier will charge $2.00 per pound. The pork loin's cold storage costs are 12 percent of the pork's value. Below are examples of EOQ calculation using the above example:

$$\sqrt{\frac{2 \times \$2.00 \times 10,542}{0.15}} = \$530.21$$

$$\sqrt{\frac{2 \times \$2.00 \times 10,542}{(\$2.25 \times .15)}} = 353.5 \text{ or } 354 \text{ lbs}$$

These calculations indicate that the most cost effective order quantity (EOQ) is $530.21 worth of pork loin, or 354 pounds of pork loin for the designated ordering period. Operations may use this information to further calculate the total annual ordering costs and storage costs for pork loin. The following equation is used:

$$\text{Total annual costs} = \frac{\text{ordering cost per order} \times \text{number of units used in one year}}{\text{order size (in units)}} + \frac{\text{storage cost per year of one unit} \times \text{order size (in units)}}{2}$$

$$\text{Total annual costs} = \frac{\$2.00 \times 10{,}542 \text{ lb}}{354 \text{ lb}} + \frac{\$2.25 \times 0.15 \times 354 \text{ lb}}{2} = \$119.30$$

These values are used by management to determine if 354 pounds of pork loin is an appropriate order size for the operation. They also help to identify the reorder point (ROP), or the number of units the on-hand item decreases before reordering. It is common that purchasers who use EOQ calculations also utilize "just in time" (JIT) inventory management. Just in time management is the practice in which items are ordered and received just in time for production use. This management allows the most desirable inventory level to be maintained at all times.

Forecasting Food Demand
Forecasting food demand is crucial to prevent overproduction. The sales forecast is the simplest method for controlling production costs. The sales forecast is found by multiplying the average check per person by the total customer count. This figure estimates the total revenue for a given period, and therefore identifying a budget for that same given period. In order to calculate the average check per person, several items must be considered. Appetizers, entrees, beverages, and desserts must be estimated for each customer. Multiplying the average appetizer price by the forecasted percentage of customers ordering appetizers will give the average check appetizer. For example, if the average cost of an appetizer is $7.50 and is ordered by 18% of customers, the average check appetizer is $1.35.

$7.50 × 1.8 = $1.35
Price × Forcast = average check

Ordering Food and Supplies
Once a vendor has been selected and food and product specifications have been identified, food and supply ordering should be on a fairly regular schedule to ensure proper ingredients and supplies are available for production in proper quantities that reduce spoilage or waste. Typically, an establishment will have a designated manager who orders food and other products. Ordering methods are different at each distributor and for each contract with the foodservice operation. Establishing proper ordering procedures will reduce inconsistencies in orders.

Food Production, Distribution, and Service

Production

The production of food involves many components that require identified policies and procedures to produce a consistent product.

Procedures
Recipes
A standardized recipe is one that has been adapted and tested to guarantee it will produce a product consistently each time it is used. Standardized recipes ensure the same food item is produced despite

being prepared by various people, the yield is predictable, the nutrient profile is accurate, and purchasing food items involves low labor.

The goal of a standardized recipe is to foster consistency. Standardized recipes should contain the following:

- Name of recipe unique and descriptive of the recipe
- Recipe category and number if applicable
- Recipe yield
- Serving size
- Ingredients
- Proper temperature measures
- Directions for preparation
- Pan or dish size, shape, and material
- Cook time
- Serving utensils

Recipes should be organized in categories that are easily maintained and understood by those using them. There are various methods to organizing recipes, which could be based on the primary ingredient, the type of dish, or meal to be served, among others. For example, a Chicken Parmesan dish may be categorized as an Italian dish, chicken dish, or dinner entrée. Nevertheless, the method adopted by the specific operation should be consistent with all recipes that exist in their recipe pool.

Scaling a recipe is an important step in cooking enough food while minimizing food waste. Recipe scaling involves adjusting a recipe to meet the needs of the operation. Scaling up is necessary when a recipe yields a smaller amount than needed, while scaling down is required when the recipe calls for more servings than desired. In order to scale a recipe up or down, a conversion factor must first be determined. For example, to scale a recipe that yields 6 servings to 125, the desired serving size is divided by the servings yielded in the original recipe (125/6) = 20.8. In order to ensure the recipe yields enough for 125, it is necessary to round up, in this case to 21. Next, the measurement for each ingredient is multiplied by 21. So, if the original recipe called for 2.5 cups of flour, the scaled up recipe needs 52.5 cups of flour (21 x 2.5). Ingredients like olive oil or butter to sauté or grease a pan generally do not need to be multiplied by as large a number.

Cooking Methods
Once food is received and stored properly, preparation to cook foods according to the standardized recipes can begin. First, frozen food must be thawed using proper procedures; food should not be thawed at room temperature due to an increased risk of foodborne microorganism growth. There are four acceptable techniques to prevent bacterial growth:

1. Food can be thawed in a refrigerator whose temperature is 41°F or below. This method may take more than one day if the food product is large.

2. Food can be submerged under running drinking water whose temperature is 70°F or lower. The pressure of the running water must remove loose food particles from food. The sink, counter, and other work areas should be sanitized before and after thawing food using this method.

The minimum internal temperature varies from food to food and may even vary from operation to operation; however, the table below lists the minimum internal cooking temperatures and the amount of time that temperature should be held for.

Product	Minimum Internal Cooking Temperatures
Poultry (chicken, turkey, duck)	165°F for 15 seconds
Stuffing and stuffed meat, poultry, fish, and pasta	165°F for 15 seconds
Temperature sensitive food cooked in a microwave (eggs, poultry, fish, and meat)	165°F
Ground meat (pork, beef, turkey, chicken)	155°F for 15 seconds
Injected meat (including brined ham and roasts)	155°F for 15 seconds
Mechanically tenderized meat	155°F for 15 seconds
Beef, lamb, pork, veal	Steaks/Chops: 145°F for 15 seconds Roasts: 145°F for 4 minutes
Seafood (crustaceans, fish, shellfish)	145°F for 15 seconds
Shell eggs for immediate service	144°F for 15 seconds
Ready-to-Eat food, commercially processed	135°F

Menu items that include raw or undercooked foods must be noted.

Most foods are prepared at the temperature listed in the table above. Because of the way it is processed, poultry has the highest counts and types of microorganisms of meats. Cooking poultry thoroughly to the minimum internal temperature of 165°F is crucial.

Produce may be consumed raw; however, cooked fruits or vegetables should be cooked to minimum internal temperature of 135°F. Cooked fruits and vegetables should be refrigerated immediately after use and should never be held at room temperature.

Foods that are temperature-controlled for safety that are reheated in a microwave require special considerations, because food is often heated unevenly in microwaves.

- To prevent the surface from drying out, the food should be covered.
- Food should be stirred or rotated halfway through cooking to circulate heat more evenly.
- Covered food should stand in microwave for two minutes, allowing for the temperature to balance.

Temperature measures of food reheated in a microwave should be done in multiple places to ensure the food is cooked throughout.

Operations may cook food partially during preparation and then finish cooking it right before service. This technique is often used in circumstances where large volumes of food are needed for service. The following guidelines should be followed when partially cooking eggs, meat, poultry, seafood, or dishes with these items:

- During initial cooking, food should not be cooked for longer than sixty minutes.
- Immediately after initial cooking, the food should be cooled.
- Cooled food should be frozen or refrigerated.
- During the second cooking period, food should be heated to at least 165°F before service.
- Food not being served immediately should be held for service at proper temperatures or cooled.

Operations may be required to present written procedures of partial cooking during preparation to local authorities for approval. Written procedures often include the following:

- Monitoring and documenting methods of procedures
- Corrective action if procedures not followed
- Identification of foods that need further cooking
- Storage solutions for partial cooked foods independent of ready-to-eat foods

Ingredient Control
Ingredient control not only protects against allergens and cross-contamination, but also theft of inventory and products. Each of these concerns can majorly affect a kitchen budget. Ordering, receiving, and storage must be well tracked and documented in order to link the system to a consumer's dietary needs. Ingredients should be stored in a labeled, organized fashion so as to not mistake ingredients for another.

Portion Control
The operation's standardized recipe determines the amount of food per serving, or portion control. The menu item may list the portion size (i.e. 6 oz. filet). The portion control not only is a main cost control for the institution, but also a key component in customers evaluating the value of the menu item. If the portion is too large, the operation may lose money due to higher food costs. On the contrary, if the product is under-portioned, the consumer may be unsatisfied and not return. Proper portioning by the operation's associates is imperative in providing consistency to all customers and in keeping food costs down.

Identifying the yield analysis for each standardized recipe provides insight into how much is needed for service. The total amount to prepare should be extracted from the day's anticipated sales for that particular menu item, combined with the yield analysis. Many tools aid in the portioning process of food including scoops, serving spoons, ladles, serving dishes, and portion scales. Scoops can be used to portion semisolid food items like ice cream, tuna salad, and cookie dough. Scoops are sized and numbered from four to forty corresponding to how many scoops the size yields per quart. For example, a number twelve yields twelve portions per quart. Scoops only provide exact portions when the product is level with the top of the scoop. Serving spoons can be slotted or solid. Slotted spoons are generally used for food items in liquid that should be served without the liquid, such as canned vegetables. Solid serving spoons are used for semisolid foods like coleslaw or mashed potatoes. One slightly rounded serving spoon typically yields four ounces. Liquids such as soups, salad dressings, sauces, and stews are portioned using a ladle. Ladles range in size from one-half ounce to eight ounces. While serving utensils are often thought of as portioning tools, serving dishes may also be used. For example, ramekins used for sauces vary from one to four ounces. Also, individual casserole dishes can contain weight to ten ounces of food. Cups and bowls also are used for portioning soups and beverages. Lastly, portion scales use weight to portion meats and other side dishes by weight.

Beverages must also have standardized portions to control beverage costs and ensure a profit. Portion control devices for beverages include jiggers and shot glasses. Portion control spouts on bottles pour a certain measurement, minimizing portion distortion by bartenders.

It is evident when cooking that some portion of the food is lost during preparation. The as purchased (AP) price is the price of an item when it comes through the door at delivery; however, many food items like fresh produce or meat are trimmed, chopped, or cooked during preparation and before serving. When ordering food items, the edible portion price must be considered. The edible portion (EP) price is the cost of an item after all trimming and assembly is done before cooking. The as served (AS) price is the cost of an item when it is served to the consumer. The AS price is comprised of food costs plus labor costs during preparation. In order to calculate the EP cost, an operation must know the AP price and the edible yield percentage. Using the previous example of pork loin, the AP price per pound is $2.25. The edible yield percentage formerly stated is 75 percent.

$$\text{EP per product unit} = \text{AP price} \div \text{Edible yield percentage}$$

$$\text{EP per product unit} = \$2.25 \div 0.75 = \$3.00$$

The EP cost of a product can also be computed on a per-serving basis using the item's AP price and portion divider (PD) that was figured as part of determining the correct order size.

$$\text{EP per serving} = \text{AP price} \div \text{PD}$$

$$\text{EP per serving} = \$2.25 \div 3 = \$0.75$$

The standard serving cost of a meal option on the menu can then be determined once the EP per serving of all components of the meal are calculated. For example, the pork loin is served with mixed vegetables (EP per-serving cost of $0.15) and a baked potato (EP per-serving cost of $0.34).

$$\text{EP cost per serving (pork loin)} + \text{EP cost per serving (baked potato)}$$
$$+ \text{EP cost per serving (vegetables)} = \text{standard cost (for pork loin meal)}$$

$$\$0.75 + \$0.34 + \$0.15 = \$1.24$$

The total standard cost of the pork loin meal is $1.24. Once the standard cost is determined, the menu costs can be created. The managers, chefs, and owners of the operation will collaborate to establish the menu prices dependent on the standard cost.

$$\text{menu price} = \text{standard cost} \div \text{percentage of menu price}$$

For example, the managers, chefs, and owners determine the pork loin meal standard cost is 30 percent of its menu price. To determine the menu price of the pork loin meal, the calculation below is computed.

$$\$1.24 \div 0.30 = \$4.13$$

The recommended food cost to the customer is the menu price of $4.13. This may be decided as the menu price; however, market conditions or competitive pricing may alter the price that is more desirable to the customer. The standard cost allows an operation to know how much it costs to produce that specific meal for the customer.

Production Systems

Some characteristics of foodservice separate it from the production of other products. These characteristics include:

- Food demand occurs at peak times (breakfast, lunch, and dinner). Slow times occur in between meals.

- The time of year may cause variance in the demand for food; production must be adapted accordingly.

- Food preparation and service are labor intensive.

- Food must be handled correctly at all points during preparation and production.

Menus may change daily, altering production demands daily.

Conventional

Conventional foodservice systems involve food production onsite, then holding it either heated or chilled, and then serving it to the consumer. Some food items may be purchased and require full preparation, while others may be purchased with minimal prep needed or even fully prepared. This type of production system can be found in schools, hospitals, colleges and universities, and restaurants. Advantages of a conventional production system include:

- High level of perceived quality by consumers, due to fresh and homemade food products
- Flexibility in menu items because food is prepped and served soon after production
- Food is served soon after production, reducing freezing, chilling, or reheating processes that may impact the quality of the food
- Standardized recipes can be used due to low incidence of chilling and reheating foods

Disadvantages also exist in the conventional production system:

- It is labor intensive. Food preparation is timed in relation to the service of food. Peaks and valleys of food demand affect a conventional system more than any other production system. Increased labor should be scheduled during peak times, consequently making labor costs highest for conventional systems compared to other systems.

- Consistency may be compromised. For example, there may be multiple conventional kitchens within a school system, resulting in a greater chance of variability in food quality, portion sizes, and food costs related to unskilled labor. A cook may decide to be creative and add more spices to a recipe, or another cook may have better cooking skills than others in the school system. All of these factors may lead to inconsistencies.

- Food costs may be higher, due to less control of portion sizes and wastes may be greater.

- Food safety is less controllable in a conventional system compared to other food service systems. In a conventional system, various employees at a number of locations must make more decisions at critical control points, making it difficult to supervise every decision.

Commissary

Commissary production systems centralize food production in one location and then transport food to satellite kitchens where it is served to consumers. Food is usually purchased unprepared and food preparation is completed in the central kitchen. Having the majority of deliveries to one location lowers food costs. Labor costs also are minimized due to one central kitchen. When mass food production is needed, the commissary foodservice system is best utilized. Once food preparation in the central kitchen is complete, it must be transported to the satellite kitchens. The temperature and packaging of the food is an important factor in commissary style productions. In order to avoid food-borne illnesses, foods must either be transported hot or cold at proper temperatures, so proper equipment must be available not only at the receiving location, but also during the transportation phase. Food may be sent in bulk or pre-plated. Proper coordination of food production and delivery schedules must occur between the central and satellite kitchens. A variety of settings utilize a commissary food system including airlines, school systems, hospitals, and restaurants.

Advantages of commissary foodservice systems:

- Lower food and supply costs. When purchasing food in very large quantities, food costs may be lower in larger quantities compared to ordering separately for several smaller operations.

- Purchasing power is increased when ordering larger quantities. Supplier or vendor issues like delivery schedules, order size, quality control, and return policies may be reduced. Items such as bread, milk, or paper products may still be delivered to the individual satellite kitchens.

- USDA commodities are used more effectively at a central location compared to several smaller kitchens. Schools often receive free government commodities. With a central kitchen, the commodities can be used more efficiently in recipes.

- Ingredient control is improved with one central kitchen. Food costs are then decreased with greater control over ingredients.

- Inventory is better controlled in a central kitchen. A process is in place to identify when inventory is ordered, how to rotate inventory to avoid spoilage, and overall maintain the quality of food.

- Labor costs can be reduced significantly using commissary systems because the overall number of employees is fewer compared to conventional foodservice systems. Producing high quantities in one location allows for higher productivity among employees.

- Food preparation scheduling is flexible if food is transported chilled. Peaks and valleys of food demand by customers is eliminated and labor costs can be better controlled. Because production is separated from service, food production can be scheduled at any time during the day.

- Quality control in the food being served is increased in a commissary foodservice system due to the central location of production. Quality control includes microbiological quality, aesthetic quality, and nutritional quality.

- Consistency is a major advantage to a commissary system. Consistency in aesthetic quality and nutritional quality is extremely important in meeting consumers' expectations.

- Flexibility in location is possible with the central kitchen. For example, if the service locations are in high-priced land areas, it may be extremely costly to build a kitchen on the land. Because food is transported to satellite kitchens in a commissary system, the central kitchen can be in a cheaper area.

- Fully equipped kitchens are not needed in each service location saving on equipment costs. This savings includes less equipment to be repaired in the future.

Disadvantages of commissary foodservice systems:

- High initial investment is needed to build and equip a central production kitchen.

- Employees with technical skills are required to produce food in large quantities.

- Some jobs may lack variety, especially when an assembly line is utilized in a commissary system.

- Equipment repair is more costly in a central production facility than in a smaller kitchen. Preventative maintenance should be utilized to reduce risk of equipment failure.

- Transporting food to the receiving kitchens requires trucks or vans and delivery equipment (gasoline, carts, insurance, maintenance and repair) that are significant expenses. Drivers may also need a Commercial Driver's License.

- Low level of perceived quality by consumers. Mass production of food is often less desirable for consumers than made-to-order food.

- Recipe modification may be required when making such large quantities. Products that are chilled or frozen may need recipe modification to maintain product quality. Standardized recipes should be retested when used in central production.

- Food safety problems may affect more customers. If there is a food-borne illness from an ingredient in the recipe, more consumers will be affected, due to the mass production of the food product.

- Employees involved in food production are not serving food to the customers. There is not an opportunity for cooks to receive direct feedback from customers regarding the quality and taste of food. Customers often seem less real to cooks, which may diminish the quality of work by the cooks.

Ready Prepared
In a ready prepared foodservice production system, food is first prepped and cooked onsite. The food is then chilled or frozen until reheated for service onsite. Food production can occur at any time of day since it is not served immediately, and multiple days of food can be prepared at once. For example, if chicken noodle soup is on the menu multiple times in the next thirty days, the total amount of chicken noodle soup for all days can be done at once, reducing labor costs. Food items may be purchased and require full preparation, while other food items need none. Hospitals and prisons are popular institutions utilizing ready prepared production systems.

Advantages of ready prepared foodservice systems include:

- Flexibility in scheduling food preparation because food is prepared ahead of time.

- Lower labor costs results when large quantities of food are prepared at one time and stored for later use.

Possible disadvantages of ready prepared foodservice systems include:

- Menu items may be limited due to foods not suitable for chilling or freezing and then reheating.

- Initial capital investment for equipment is high; however, lower food and labor costs often offset the initial costs in a short period of time.

- Low level of perceived quality by consumers. Mass production of food is often less desirable for consumers than made-to-order food.

- Recipe modifications may be necessary due to large quantities produced and the cooling, freezing, and reheating processes. Food quality must be upheld in the production of large quantities.

- Food safety issues affect more consumers since food items are made in bulk. Tight controls and policies should be in place to reduce risk of food-borne illness.

Assembly Serve
Assembly serve foodservice systems involve purchasing food that needs little to no preparation. Food can be stored frozen or chilled to then later be portioned out, reheated, and served to consumers.

Advantages of assembly serve foodservice systems include:

- Lower labor costs are a result from purchasing foods needing little to no preparation for service.

- Equipment needs are also low because the food is purchased premade. Most menu items only need reheating and portioning before service. This minimal preparation requires minimal equipment.

Disadvantages of assembly serve foodservice systems:

- High food cost due to foods being purchased with little to no preparation needed.

- Limited menu variety compared to convention, commissary, or ready prepared because menu items are restricted to those available pre-made.

- Availability of menu items in a cyclic menu may not continue to be available because food companies have discontinued that product or the distributor no longer carries that specific product.

- Low level of perceived quality by consumers. Mass production of food is often less desirable for consumers than made-to-order food.

Cook-Chill

The cook-chill foodservice production system is designed to provide flexibility in the time of preparation of food. Food is first fully cooked followed by rapid chilling and storage at controlled temperatures for up to five days. When appropriate, food must be reheated to proper temperatures before service. Cook-chill is most common in large institutional foodservice operations; however, smaller and more compact equipment is now available for small to medium-sized operations to use.

Advantages of cook-chill foodservice systems include:

- Time is used more efficiently. Most cooking can take place outside of peak hours, leaving more time to serve customers effectively.

- Resources are used more effectively, as food can be made for multiple operations in one kitchen.

- Selection of menu items is more extensive because a greater selection of menu items can be prepared ahead of time.

- Modification of recipes is generally not necessary in a cook-chill foodservice system.

- Because food is prepared ahead of time, faster service can be provided to customers.

- Waste is reduced and portion control is improved because food can be reheated as heated.

- In a cook-chill foodservice system, an operation can offer a wide variety of menu items to a large number of customers in a short amount of time. This opportunity gives an operation a chance for increased profitability.

Display Cooking

A production system featuring display cooking is a more recent trend in the restaurant business. The preparation and cooking of menu items is visible to the consumer. This type of production system is popular in high-end restaurants, but also in some fast-casual restaurants. The benefit of having the preparation and cooking process on display for the consumers is that it can give the consumer comfort in seeing the food they will eat being prepared. The customer may also find comfort in the cleanliness of the kitchen, and be familiar with whoever is preparing the menu items. Disadvantages that exist in a display cooking production system revolve around the pressure of presentation for the kitchen and staff. The kitchen and staff are on display, so the kitchen must be well kept at all times, and staff members must be a suitable representation for the establishment.

Distribution and Service

Form of Food Delivered

Delivery of food requires proper temperatures to be maintained to avoid bacteria growth that may result in foodborne illness. Temperatures must avoid the danger zone of 41°F to 140°F. If being served immediately after delivery, temperatures should be maintained during course of delivery and eaten within two hours. If food will be served at a later time, the delivered food must be refrigerated at 40°F or below and at 0°F or below if frozen.

Type of Service Systems

A centralized food service system involves food that is prepared near or in the same production area in which the completed food order is delivered or served to consumers. Centralized delivery-service systems require close supervision to maintain food quality and control portion sizes. Examples of institutions using a centralized delivery-service system are fast food restaurants, banquet services, hospitals, and long-term care facilities.

On the contrary, decentralized delivery-service systems prepare bulk quantities of food that is then sent hot or cold to satellite kitchens or serving kitchenettes located throughout the facility. If necessary, portioning, reheating, and meal assembly take place in the remote serving locations. Serving utensils and dishes are returned to the central kitchen for washing. Decentralized delivery-service systems are appropriate in institutions where there is a large distance between the kitchen and consumer like large hospitals, school districts, medical centers, university campuses, hotels, and resorts.

Clients and Customers Served

Understanding the clientele of the restaurant is crucial in meeting the expectations to provide appropriate service and ensure customers will return to the establishment. The ambiance and environment should match the service given to customers. White tablecloths and linen napkins would suggest service to the table, whereas a fast-casual restaurant may require walk-up ordering and retrieval of food. If customers are expected to remove dishes from the table, there should be multiple easy-to-get-to areas for them to do so.

Schedules of Assembly and Breakdown

The managerial staff should create a schedule of the assembly of food and the breakdown of food at the end of service. Food should not be held at proper temperatures for longer than two hours. If food still remains after two hours, it should be discarded. During breakdown, food that that can be saved and chilled for reuse should be placed in containers with a secure lid or sealed plastic wrap.

Room Service

Room service in a hospital, long-term care facility, or hotel allows the customer to order food or beverage items off of a menu from the comfort of his or her room and have it delivered at a specified time. When food and beverage is traveling from the kitchen to the destination, it must be covered and remain at adequate temperatures. The travel time and distance must not be too long or far to promote menu items entering the temperature danger zone.

Physical and Chemical Properties of Food

Meat, Poultry, and Fish

Muscle is composed of bundles of fibers called myofibrils. Connective tissue surrounding the myofibrils contains collagen and elastin and holds the fibers in the bundles. In the presence of heat, collagen is hydrolyzed to gelatin and becomes tender. Elastin is cartilage, yellow in color, and changes very little during the cooking process. Fat is deposited around organs and muscles. Meat, poultry and fish contain 16 percent to 23 percent protein, carbohydrates, some vitamins and trace minerals. Most fish have less fat and fewer calories than meat but still provide a good dietary source of protein. Myoglobin in meat contributes to the color. When first exposed to oxygen, meat turns red, and further exposure turns it brown, and then green.

Eggs

The color of the eggshell has no influence of the flavor or quality of the egg. The interior, near either pole, contains an air space that becomes larger with age. The egg yolk is a naturally occurring oil-in-water emulsion. Eggs contain approximately 80 calories, 6 grams of protein, 5 grams of fat, vitamins A, D, and riboflavin. The yolk contains more protein by weight than the white and has a greater concentration of fat, vitamins, and minerals. The hen's diet will influence the color of the yolk. Egg size (jumbo, extra large, large, medium, or small) is based on the weight per dozen. A fresh egg will sink to the bottom of a pan of cold water and has a dull shell. In cooking, eggs provide structure and stability and are used as binding agents.

The albumin (egg white) is a high quality protein that contains all of the essential amino acids. It is also a good source of niacin, riboflavin, potassium, and magnesium. The egg yolk, while the source of cholesterol and fat, contains vitamin A, vitamin D, vitamin E, and zinc.

Milk and Dairy
Milk is a good source of calcium, phosphorus, riboflavin, vitamins A and D, but is low in iron. It is approximately 87% water, 3.5% protein (which contains far more casein than whey), up to 3.7% fat, and 4.9% carbohydrate (lactose). Homogenization breaks down fat globules. Pasteurization destroys pathogenic bacteria. Vitamin D can be added by directly injecting the vitamin, exposing it to ultraviolet light, or by increasing the amount of vitamin D in the cow's diet. Two percent milk may contain up to 2.25% milk fat, 1% (low-fat) milk may contain up to 2% milk fat, while fat free (skim) must contain no more than 0.5% milk fat. Evaporated milk has had 60% of the water removed. Sweetened condensed milk is evaporated whole milk with added sugar. Buttermilk is made by adding lactic acid bacteria to skimmed or partially skimmed milk. Sweet acidophilus milk is skim milk with the addition of acidophilus bacteria, which reduces the lactose content. Kefir is milk fermented by Lactobacillus kefir, which adds carbon dioxide and a small amount of alcohol. Low-lactose milk (such as the brand name Lactaid) is treated with lactase (enzyme responsible for breaking down lactose) during processing. Yogurt is coagulated milk that has been fermented by lactic acid bacteria. Some yogurt brands may have other cultures added to them.

Most milk and milk products sold in the United States are pasteurized, though there is growing interest in the sale and purchase of raw milk and milk products. Milk is pasteurized to destroy pathogens harmful to humans and extend shelf life by destroying the bacteria that causes spoilage. Ultra-high temperature processing (UHT) heats a product in excess of boiling and renders it sterile. This creates a product with a shelf life of six months or longer, but can also influence the flavor.

Homogenization is an emulsification process that suspends small fat globules in liquid layer. The reduced surface area of the fat globules allows them to stay suspended in the liquid layer and stabilizes the emulsion.

Vegetables and Fruit
Vegetables and fruit may contain between 75% and 93% water. They are also a source of both soluble and insoluble fiber, some minerals, and vitamins such as C and A. They contain hemicellulose and lignin. Lignin is responsible for providing structure in plants. During ripening and storage, enzymes are responsible for the conversion of starch to sugar. Pectin is converted to pectic acid and is responsible for the properties of overripe fruit. Ethylene gas is naturally given off by certain fruits such as apples and accelerates ripening during storage. Chlorophyll is green, carotenoids are yellow and orange, anthocyanins are red, blue, purple, and lycopenes contribute red color and act as antioxidants, while anthoxanthins or flavones are white. Carotenoids are least affected by the pH of a cooking solution. Chlorophyll will turn olive green in acid and bright green in an alkaline solution. Acids, sugar, and aromatic compounds contribute to the flavor of fruit.

Flour
Whole grain flour is made with the entire grain and can spoil quickly due to the fat contents of the germ. Bread flour (or hard wheat) contains the most protein and strong gluten. All-purpose flour (a blend of

soft and hard wheat) has less gluten and contains approximately 10.5% protein. Pastry flour (soft wheat) contains weaker gluten and approximately 7.9% protein. Cake flour is the softest and contains the least and weakest gluten, the least amount of protein, and high starch content. Self-rising flour is a blend of flour, baking powder, and salt. Durum wheat flour is high in gluten. Semolina flour is made by removing the bran and germ and grinding the starch. Flours are enriched with thiamin, riboflavin, niacin, iron, and folic acid and have become an important source of these nutrients in the typical American diet. Gluten in flour gives products elastic properties, structure, and holds in leavening agents.

Fats and Oils
Oils are liquid at room temperature. Sources of oils include plants, nuts, and fish. The majority of oils are high in monounsaturated or polyunsaturated fats and low in saturated fats. Coconut oil, palm kernel oil, and palm oil are high in saturated fat. Plant sources of oil such as canola, olive, and soy do not contain any cholesterol. They provide essential nutrients such as Omega-3 fats. Foods made mainly of oil include salad dressings, mayonnaise, and soft margarines. Fats that are solid at room temperature such as shortening and butter are derived from animal products and contain saturated fat. Lard and oil are 100% fat, while margarine is only about 80% fat. Other animal fats used in cooking include pork fat or lard, chicken fat, beef fat or tallow, and milk fat. Adding fat to baked products contributes to tenderness or flakiness. Fat contributes flavor to savory dishes.

Engineered Foods
Also known as genetically engineered foods, engineered foods are created when one food has the genes from other plants or animals inserted into its genetic code. Genetic engineering is accomplished with plants, animals, bacteria or other microorganisms. Proponents of engineered foods state that the food created may be more nutritious, more resistant to disease and drought, may reduce the use of pesticides, and create faster growing plants and animals. Opponents of engineered foods state that modified plants or animals may breed with natural plants or animals causing unknown environmental effects, plants may become less resistance to some pests, and genetic changes may cause harmful effects on animals or people that eat them.

Functional Foods
Functional foods have been shown to provide greater nutritional benefits. Some functional foods are naturally occurring while others are created by fortifying other substances. Some margarines have plant sterols and esters added, with the goal of reducing LDL cholesterol. Resveratrol, found in grape juice and red wine, has been shown to reduce platelet aggregation. Yogurts are cultured with different strains of bacteria to promote gastrointestinal health. Lycopene, found in tomatoes, has been shown to reduce the risk of prostrate cancer in men. Soluble fiber, found in oatmeal, can lower cholesterol.

Food Preparation

Functions of Ingredients
Ingredients in foods contribute to color, structure, taste, shelf stability, freeze/thaw properties, and nutritional value.

Techniques and Methods
Bake: dry heat preparation achieved by using an oven

Baste: the process of adding moisture, flavor, and color to foods by brushing, spooning, or drizzling pan juices or sauces over the food during the cooking process

Blackened: method in which food is generally heavily seasoned and cooked over high heat until charred

Boil: cooking in liquid that is heated until it bubbles

Broil: the use of radiated heat

Braise: cooking slowly in a small amount of liquid while covered

Brown: food cooked typically in fat or oil until the surface turns brown in color; does not usually cook food completely and is the first step in a longer cooking process. It often occurs on a hot pan or under the broiler and is meant to seal in juices and flavor.

Chop: cutting food into small, uniform pieces; can be accomplished with a knife or food processor

Clarify: the process of skimming fat from the surface of a liquid (such as melted butter)

Cream: the process of mixing butter or another fat until fluffy; this is sometimes done with another ingredient such as sugar

Cut-in: combining a solid fat (lard, shortening, or butter) with dry ingredients until small crumb-like pieces are formed. The fat is usually pre-chilled and is cut-in with a pastry cutter, fork, or fingers.

Deglaze: the process of making a sauce or gravy in which a small amount of liquid is added to a hot pan that was used to cook a protein. As the liquid heats, the pan is scraped to remove small browned bits from the pan to incorporate them into the sauce or gravy.

Dissolve: the process of mixing a solid into a liquid to form a homogenous solution

Dredge: to coat a food with flour or bread crumbs; often done before frying

Fold: the process of gently mixing ingredients to prevent over-beating or flattening; usually done with a rubber spatula in a downward sweeping and across motion

Fry: cooking or browning in oil quickly, at high temperatures

Garnish: an object (such as an herb, flower, or sauce) used to dress a plate. Can also refer to the action of dressing the plate

Grease: coating a pan with a layer of fat prior to cooking or baking to prevent food from sticking to the pan

Julienne: cutting food into thin strips that are approximately the size of a match

Knead: the process of folding and pressing down on dough until a smooth texture is achieved. This process activates the gluten, which results in a cohesive product.

Macerate: soaking fruits or vegetables in a liquid or sugar, which causes the food to soften and enhance its flavor

Marinate: soaking a protein in a liquid and spices to tenderize it and/or add flavor

Mince: chopping food into very small pieces, usually irregular in shape and size

Pare: using a knife or peeler to peel the skin from a fruit or vegetable

Poach: cooking food in simmering water or another liquid

Preheat: turning on an oven or other cooking device to allow it to rise to the appropriate temperature prior to heating the food

Puree: blending a food using a blender, food processor, stick blender, or other device until it becomes a thick liquid. Also the term applied to the liquid.

Reduce: allowing the water to cook off or evaporate from a sauce, causing it to thicken and intensify in flavor

Roasting: cook in oven, often at low temperatures to prevent a tough finished product

Render: to remove the fat from a protein by cooking, heating, and/or straining

Sauté: the use of a small amount of hot oil to heat and brown foods in an open pan over high heat, turning and tossing it

Score: lightly cutting the surface of a food prior to cooking it, often to allow flavors to penetrate the surface

Sear: utilized to trap flavors and juices in a protein by quickly browning it on all sides before cooking to the final temperature

Shred: cutting food into small, thin strips by using a grating surface or by hand chopping, or to pull apart tender meat with a fork after cooking

Simmer: cooking in water or another liquid gently just below boiling point

Steam: heat over, not in, water

Stewing: add water or other liquid during cooking in a covered pot or pan

Toss: a method to combine foods by lightly lifting and dropping the foods; usually done in a large bowl

Whip: mixing method, usually with a whisk, fork, blender, or stand mixer, in which food is mixed in a quick and light fashion to incorporate air into the food or mixture

Effects on Food Quality
Dry heat cooking methods (frying, broiling, grilling, and roasting) are best suited for cuts of meats with less connective tissue. Connective tissue can be difficult to soften and break down and if not cooked properly will contribute to a dry, tough dish. Moist heat cooking methods (stewing, simmering, braising, steaming) allows the connective tissue to gelatinize and therefore tenderize the meat. More expensive cuts of meat tend to have less connective tissue.

Effects on Nutrient Retention
Certain foods like fruits and vegetables should be cooked or heated at as low a heat as possible for the shortest amount of time as possible to prevent the nutrients from seeping out into the cooking liquid. Steaming or microwaving vegetables is the best way to retain those nutrients.

Food Additives

Certain ingredients have very specific purposes in prepared food. BHA, BHT, and vitamin E are antioxidants and are added to foods to prevent fats from turning rancid and to prevent discoloration. Emulsifiers suspend and distribute fats in liquids and are used to improve the texture of foods like ice cream, pastries, and candy. Emulsifiers are also used in mixtures like mayonnaise to prevent separation. Humectants are often used in products like candy to maintain moisture levels, freshness, and the desired texture. Nitrates and nitrites are often added to processed meats to inhibit growth of C. botulinum. Ascorbic acid, calcium propionate, and sodium benzoate are also common preservatives. The goal of all preservatives is to inhibit microbial growth, prevent oxidation, and prevent rancidity.

Sanitation, Safety, Equipment, and Facilities

Safety

The safety of the employees and consumers is the first area of concern in any foodservice operation. Policies and procedures to increase safety should be well covered in the employee training.

Employee Safety

All employees must be well trained in order to optimize safety in the work place. Training should include but not be limited to personal hygiene, safe food prep, cleaning and sanitizing, and safe chemical handling.

Safety Programs and Practices

Proper training for employees for all aspects of the operation will help keep employees safe on the job. Depending on local laws where the institution is located, employees should be ServSafe certified or hold a Food Handler's Permit from the local authorities. In addition, operations should inform and train employees annually who use hazardous chemicals. Each operation should have a Material Safety Data Sheet (MSDS) for each hazardous chemical at the establishment. Manufacturers are required to send the MSDS forms when shipping the chemicals. The MSDS sheet must be kept in a place that is easily accessible to all employees. Employee training must also include plans in the event of fire, water leak, or other crisis to properly take action and keep themselves, other employees, and customers safe.

Customer Safety

Customer safety is a priority to an operation. Food should be prepared using proper utensils, materials, and cooked to adequate temperatures to avoid foodborne illness. The dining area, bathroom, patio, or other areas accessible to customers should not pose risk of harm. If floors are wet, wet floor signs must be in the vicinity to make customers aware. If something is out of order, a sign must indicate the issue. These areas should be monitored frequently to ensure the area remains safe throughout service.

Sanitation and Food Safety

Upholding sanitation practices in all areas of foodservice is a key component of guaranteeing that food that is consumed is safe and to reduce the risk of unwanted items in the food served, as well as a foodborne illness outbreak.

Principles

Strong principles should be in place to avoid contamination and spoilage. Employees should be properly trained and made aware of factors contributing to bacterial growth.

Contamination and Spoilage
Timetables are in place to identify the length of time that food should be kept and/or served to avoid contamination and spoilage. Dated stickers or labels are placed on foods items to note the date the food item should be disposed of or used by. Employees must be trained to understand the timeframe for various types of foods prepared by the institution.

Factors Affecting Bacterial Growth
Factors affecting bacterial growth include:

- Bacteria are mostly controlled by keeping food out of the temperature danger zone.

- Bacteria can grow rapidly if food, acidity, temperature, time, oxygen, and moisture are in proper conditions for growth.

- Some bacteria may change into a different form, called spores, to protect themselves.

- Certain bacteria produce toxins in food as they grow and die. When humans eat toxins, illness can result; toxins may or may not be killed during the cooking process.

Signs and Symptoms of Food Borne Illness
There are many signs and symptoms of food-borne illness. The most common include diarrhea, nausea, vomiting, abdominal pain, and fever. Other less common signs and symptoms are bloody diarrhea, double vision, weakness, kidney failure, sepsis, pneumonia, meningitis, and miscarriage in pregnant women.

Sanitation Practices and Infection Control
Personal hygiene should be a main concern for employees before and during their shift. Personnel must be trained on proper personal hygiene practices and food handling techniques. Training should not stop there. Employees should understand how to use equipment effectively to guarantee it is accurately maintaining food quality.

Personal Hygiene
Proper personal hygiene is crucial in the prevention of foodborne illness. Good personal hygiene includes:

- Following proper hand practices
- Keeping uniform and clothing clean
- Maintain personal hygiene
- Upholding good health
- Avoiding the workplace when ill

Food and Equipment Temperature Control
The temperature of food should be continuously checked with the correct thermometer and recorded in a temperature log. The log should be dated and include the food being measured, the time the temperature was taken, what the temperature was, and who took the temperature. Policies and procedures should be well established in the event the food does not meet temperature ranges.

Equipment must receive regular maintenance to certify it is working properly to store and cook foods to correct temperatures. Maintenance logs should be kept to document the history of the equipment. The temperature of the respective equipment should also be checked on a regular schedule and recorded in a temperature log. Procedures must be in place if equipment is not holding at the desired temperatures.

Food Handling Techniques

Once an employee's hands are washed, they may begin handling food. Single-use gloves should be worn when handling food, and discarded when soiled, beginning a different task, at least every four hours of continued use, after handling raw meat, and before handling ready-to-eat food. Ready-to-eat food should be prepared before handling raw meats if in confined areas, or away from raw meats if space allows. Cutting boards, utensils, and services must be washed and sanitized before using with new foods.

HACCP

A Hazard Analysis Critical Control Point (HACCP) system identifies biological, chemical, or physical hazards at specific points during the production of food at an operation. These identifiable points of potential hazards can then be avoided, prevented, or reduced to safe levels. There are seven principles in a HACCP plan.

- Principle 1: A hazard analysis is conducted to determine and assess potential physical, chemical, and biological hazards in the food being served.

- Principle 2: Critical control points (CCP) are determined to reduce or eliminate potential food risk.

- Principle 3: Minimum and Maximum limits should be established for each CCP to prevent or eliminate hazards.

- Principle 4: Monitoring procedures are established to ensure critical limits are within acceptable limits consistently.

- Principle 5: Corrective actions and steps to be taken when a critical limit is not met are established.

- Principle 6: Verification that the system is working. The system should be evaluated regularly to determine that the plan effectively prevents, reduces, and eliminates the identified hazards for the operation.

- Principle 7: Procedures for record keeping and documentation, as well as follow through with recording all events in the HACCP system, are established.

HACCP plans are required when preparing foods in the following methods:

- Smoking food to preserve it (not to enhance flavor)
- Using food additives so time and temperature controls for safety is no longer required
- Curing food
- Custom-processing animals
- Packaging food using reduced-oxygen methods like vacuum-packed foods
- Treating and packaging juice on site for sale later
- Sprouting beans or seeds
- Offering live shellfish from a display tank

<u>Regulations</u>
Regulations for food safety exist at the federal, state, and local levels. Within the government exists agencies focusing on certain aspects of food safety.

Governmental
In the United States, government control of food is applied at three levels: federal, state, and local. The U.S. Department of Agriculture (USDA) and the Food and Drug Administration (FDA) are involved in the inspection process at the federal level. The USDA inspects and grades meat, meat products, poultry, eggs, egg products, dairy products, and fruit and vegetables shipped across state lines. The FDA examines foodservice operations that cross state lines including interstate foodservice businesses on planes, trains, food manufacturers, and processors. The USDA and FDA both share responsibility of inspecting food-processing plants to guarantee standards are being met.

At the state level, food regulations are written that affect foodservice operations within the state. State or local (city or county) health departments may enforce food regulations. States may also adopt the *FDA Food Code* or a similar form of it. The *FDA Food Code* is issued by the FDA and lists the government's recommendations for foodservice regulations. The regulations are updated every two years. The intention of the *Code* is to guide state health departments in creating foodservice inspection programs; however, states are not required to adopt the practices.

Agencies
Many agencies at the federal government level exist to protect the sanitary quality of food in an operation. The USDA and FDA are two federal government agencies discussed above. Other agencies involved in food safety include the Centers for Disease Control and Prevention (CDC), the Environmental Protection Agency (EPA), and the National Marine Fisheries Service (NMFS).

The CDC provides the following services:

- Explores outbreaks of food-borne illness
- Examines the causes and control of disease
- Reports statistical data and case studies in the Morbidity and Mortality Weekly Report (MMWR)
- Provides educational information for sanitation
- Conducts an inspection program for cruise ships called the Vessel Sanitation Program

The EPA regulates the use of pesticides, handles wastes, and determines air- and water-quality standards.

The NMFS is an agency of the U.S. Department of Commerce. It implements an optional inspection program outfitted with product criteria and sanitary requirements for fish-processing operations.

<u>Food Quality and Safety</u>
The handling of food is extremely important in ensuring food maintains its quality while remaining safe for consumption. Ensuring foods are cooked, held, and stored at proper temperatures is crucial in both quality and safety. Food additives play a role in food quality, specifically the shelf life. Having a crisis team and plan in place in the event of an emergency will help to diffuse chaos.

Temperature
One crucial factor in ensuring the safety and quality of food is managing the temperature. When food is time-temperature abused, it is at high risk of microorganism growth. Microorganisms grow best in temperatures between 41°F and 135°F. This range is known as the temperature danger zone. The more

time that food stays in the temperature danger zone, the greater the time microorganisms have to grow and make food unsafe. If food is in the temperature danger zone for four hours or more, it must be discarded. Food must be cooked to the required minimum internal temperature, cooled and reheated properly, and held at the appropriate temperature. Procedures must be in place for employees to follow in order to avoid time-temperature abuse. A successful plan includes:

- Determining the most effective way to monitor time and temperature. This involves identifying which foods should be monitored, how often, and by whom.

- Ensuring correct instruments are available and accessible to take temperatures of food. Thermometers and timers should be in each area to take temperatures and monitor the time a food is kept in the temperature danger zone.

- Confirming that employees are regularly recording temperatures and the time the temperatures are taken. Time and temperature logs should be kept in an organized fashion to document appropriate data.

- Integrating time and temperature controls into standard operational duties for employees. These controls may be removing only the amount of food from the refrigerator or freezer that can be prepared in a short period of time, refrigerating utensils used for refrigerated items, and cooking food to stated minimum internal temperatures.

- Developing corrective action plans in the event that time and temperature standards are not met.

Additives
Food additives are added to food to lengthen its shelf life. They may also be added to alter food to reduce vulnerability to time and temperature abuse. Examples include nitrates, nitrites, and sulfites.

Documentation and Record Keeping
Documentation and record keeping is an essential aspect of having a successful foodservice operation. Records should be kept for the following:

- Monitoring activities
- Taking corrective action
- Certifying equipment (good working condition)
- Working with suppliers

Establishments should check with local authorities to determine how long records must be kept on file.

Crisis Management
Despite the training, policies, and procedures put in place, a food-borne illness outbreak or other crisis like power outage, flood, water service interruption, or fire may still occur. Responding to the crisis dictates the outcome of the scenario. A written crisis management program should be in place that focuses on three parts: preparation, response, and recovery. The resources needed and procedures to be followed should be included in the written plan. First, a multidisciplinary crisis management team should be created. The size is dependent on the size of the establishment. Areas of personnel to involve in the team may represent senior management, risk management, public relations, finance, operations, marketing, and human resources. Emergency contact lists should be available in the event of an emergency, as well as a crisis communication plan in which a designated spokesperson handles media

relations, if applicable. Lastly, a crisis kit should be prepared ahead of time and made accessible to the facility.

Once the preparation is complete, the crisis response should emulate the written crisis management plan. The following must be considered to control the crisis:

- Work with the media to ensure correct information is reported.
- Communicate information directly to all major audiences.
- Fix the issue at hand and communicate what was done to resolve the matter.

Recovery and assessment should follow the response to a crisis. In order to get the operation up and running again, it is crucial to determine what steps must be taken to guarantee the operation and foods remain safe.

Equipment and Facility Planning

Planning a new facility has numerous components to consider so that it effectively carries out the day-to-day duties of a foodservice establishment.

Layout Design and Planning Considerations
The layout design of a kitchen should allow it to be cleaned efficiently. The following elements will be addressed in the design of a kitchen:

- Work flow: the goal of an efficient workflow is to minimize the amount of time food spends in the temperature danger zone, as well as the amount of time food is handled. An example is having prep tables located near refrigerators and freezers to prevent delays in storing food.

- Contamination: a well-thought layout will reduce the risk of cross-contamination.

- Equipment accessibility: having equipment be as accessible as possible will ensure that the equipment will be cleaned regularly.

Presenting the plan to authorities for review may be mandatory but also can be beneficial to guarantee that the plan meets regulatory requirements, allows for a safe flow of food, and saves time and money for the establishment.

Roles and Responsibilities of Planning Team Members
When creating a team for a foodservice institution, hiring qualified team members is a crucial asset to running a successful operation. First, surveying what positions are needed will determine the number and type of associates needed for production. Determining the length of service time, the production schedule, and daily duties will also help to pinpoint the correct number of employees to have on staff at each time.

Someone from the management staff should be on duty at all times. Depending on the size of the operation, it may be necessary to have front of house management and back of house management.

Overall, each position must have clear descriptions formulated for what is expected from the employee in that position.

<u>Equipment Specification</u>
When creating specifications for equipment, it is necessary to not only consider the usage, but also to focus on sanitation. Surfaces that come into contact with food must be:

- Safe
- Durable
- Corrosion-resistant
- Nonabsorbent
- Ample in weight and thickness to weather repeated cleaning
- Smooth and easy to clean
- Resistant to chipping, scratching, decomposing, nicking, and pitting

<u>Equipment Selection</u>
Choosing equipment intended for sanitation has been streamlined by organizations like NSF International and Underwriters Laboratories (UL). NSF International composes and issues standards for sanitary equipment design. The NSF emblem on foodservice equipment signifies that after evaluation and testing, the equipment meets international commercial food equipment standards and is certified by NSF. UL also provides sanitation classification listings for NSF certified equipment. Additionally, UL lists products in compliance with their own published environmental and public health (EPH) standards.

When selecting equipment for a food service establishment, managers should look for the NSF International symbol or the UL EPH emblem. Only commercial foodservice equipment should be used, as household equipment is not meant to endure heavy use.

<u>Sustainability</u>
The foodservice industry can play a taxing role on the environment. It is imperative that operations analyze their day-to-day work and choose sustainable practices when possible.

Food and Water
Decreasing food waste will not only save on food and labor costs, but also on the garbage bill. Up to 10 percent of food purchases end up as pre-consumer waste from overproduction, spoilage, overcooking, incorrect orders, and vegetable trimmings. Post-consumer waste makes up an extremely large portion of an operation's waste; however, it is more difficult to control. Methods of reducing post-consumer waste for an institution include: reducing portion sizes, offering half-portions and children's menus, and ensuring the staff is properly trained and given the correct portion sizes.

Tracking waste should be a daily routine for staff members. Tracking will help to identify any trends in food waste. For example, if multiple pizzas are thrown out because they are burnt during the lunch service, those employees may need additional training on cooking pizzas. If salad lettuce is continuously discarded on Thursdays, it may be necessary to order less lettuce early in the week. This not only cuts back on waste, but also on food costs.

Water efficiency in food service operations is often poor; however, it should not deter the effort in implementing water sustainability practices. Because water is used in cooking, cleaning, and sanitary practices, it is a major aspect of foodservice. It is important to survey the entire operation to pinpoint areas to conserve water. The EPA's Watersense program rates and qualifies plumbing fixtures that are water efficient like aerators, faucets, urinals, toilets, showerheads, and landscape irrigation. Water conservation is augmented by incorporating as many qualifying fixtures that are applicable to the institution. Employee practices are also a crucial area for water sustainability. Integrating effective practices into employee training and company policies will set a standard of the operation's commitment to sustainability. Practices include:

- Defrost meats in refrigerator instead of under running water
- Keep pasta cookers at a simmer than a rapid boil
- Get a water audit from water utility
- Practice proper fat, oil, and grease handling best practices
- Serve water to consumers on request only

Non-Food

Supplies
Reusable and disposable products are used daily to run a foodservice operation. Fortunately, many products exist that are more sustainable than products used in the past, which now incorporate recycled content, biodegradable products, and reusable possibilities. Each process involved in the operation, including prepping, cooking, cleaning, and serving, should be surveyed to identify any materials that may be eliminated, reduced, or switched to an environmentally-friendly product. For example, unnecessary garnishes or decorations to drinks and dishes can be eliminated, and customers can be encouraged to bring their own reusable cup. Each institution will have multiple ways to cut down on supplies or find improved products to use to be mindful of the surrounding environment.

Equipment
Energy Star certifies equipment to ensure it uses energy efficiently. When possible, equipment purchased should be energy efficient. Not only are there benefits to the environment, but often times cash benefits are available for institutions using energy efficient appliances. Over the long term, energy bills will also be less expensive and may decrease the operation's costs. Steam cookers, dishwashers, and ice machines are three pieces of commercial kitchen equipment labeled Energy Star that also have water efficiency requirements.

Waste Management

Storage
Garbage cans must be waterproof, leak proof, pest proof, durable, and easy to clean. Garbage should be stored away from food preparation and storage areas, and must be large enough to house all garbage. Garbage containers, both inside and outside, should be incorporated on the cleaning duties of the establishment. Operations must contact local companies zoned to collect trash where the establishment is located. Specific dumpsters may need to be purchased or provided by the commercial waste company. If a dumpster is necessary, scheduling pickup days with the waste company will be required.

Reduction
The Environmental Protection Agency (EPA) recommends three tactics for managing waste:

1. Reduce the amount of waste produced by eliminating excessive packaging.

2. Reuse containers when possible. Chemical containers should never be reused as food containers. Containers must be cleaned and sanitized before reuse.

3. Recycle materials. Recyclables should be stored in a proper place where there is no risk of food or equipment contamination or attracting pests.

Disposal

Every institution must consider the important issue of waste management. First, operations must develop mechanisms to reduce garbage and reuse items when possible. Recycling and composting should also be considered for the removal of waste. It is possible that foodservice establishments will still create waste that must be disposed of in a traditional manner. Garbage is a large attractor for pests, which may not only contaminate food, but also utensils and equipment when handled improperly. Garbage should be removed from food-prep areas frequently to avoid odors and pest problems.

Garbage disposals may be used to discard food waste. Local regulations may limit the use of disposals in operations due to the stress that excessive food waste can put on the local wastewater systems.

Practice Questions

1. All but which of the following are factors measured in determining customer satisfaction?
    a. Sale trends
    b. Client feedback
    c. Employee input
    d. Implementing change

2. What is the purpose of product specifications?
    a. To illustrate the characteristics of the particular service or product, as well as how a product is purchased
    b. To identify exactly what products were necessary for a particular menu item
    c. To classify where food items would be purchased and delivered
    d. To determine what non-food items were required for preparation and service

3. Before product specifications are created, what must first be established?
    a. Menu items
    b. Quality standards of the restaurant
    c. Service hours
    d. Restaurant staff

4. What governmental agency provides quality measurements or indicators of eggs, poultry, and beef for consumers?
    a. Food and Drug Administration (FDA)
    b. Academy of Nutrition and Dietetic (AND)
    c. United States Department of Agriculture (USDA)
    d. Center for Food Safety and Applied Nutrition (CDSAN)

5. The place of origin of a product indicates exactly where a food item is coming from. Why is the place of origin significant?
    a. The menu may state that an ingredient is from a certain region
    b. The flavor and texture of food may vary from region to region
    c. Operations may market serving local food to guarantee quality
    d. All of the above

6. What is the goal of a procurement process?
    a. Identify policies and procedures for ordering, receiving, and storing of goods
    b. Create a training program for employees
    c. Establish daily food prep duties
    d. Determine how many staff members are needed during service

7. What is a recipe that has been adapted and tested to guarantee a consistent product called?
    a. Consistent recipe
    b. Standardized recipe
    c. Perfect recipe
    d. Complete recipe

8. All but which of the following are acceptable techniques to prevent bacteria growth?
    a. Thaw food in a refrigerator with a temperature of 41°F or lower.
    b. Submerge food under running drinking water whose temperature is 70°F or below.
    c. Thaw in the microwave if going to be used at a later time.
    d. Thaw food as part of the cooking process.

9. All but which of the following steps should be taken to limit the risk of food-borne illness?
    a. Work area, cutting boards, and utensils should be cleaned and sanitized before use.
    b. All foods and ingredients in a recipe should be prepared at the same time to ensure continuity of prep.
    c. Hands should be washed often and properly.
    d. Raw meat should be prepared in a different work area than fresh produce.

10. Which of the following is not a temperature control safety (TCS) food?
    a. Eggs
    b. Chicken salad
    c. Potato salad
    d. Cottage cheese

11. What is the as purchased (AP) price?
    a. The cost of an item after trimming and assembly is done
    b. The price the food item is sold to the consumer
    c. The cost of the menu item before it is marked up for profit
    d. The cost of an item when it comes through the door at delivery

12. What is the edible portion (EP) price?
    a. The cost of an item after trimming and assembly is done
    b. The price the food item is sold to the consumer
    c. The cost of the menu item before it is marked up for profit
    d. The cost of an item when it comes through the door at delivery

13. What is the as served (AS) price?
    a. The cost of an item after trimming and assembly is done
    b. The price the food item is sold to the consumer
    c. The cost of the menu item before it is marked up for profit
    d. The cost of an item when it comes through the door at delivery

14. What is a characteristic of a conventional foodservice system?
    a. Food production is centralized in one location and then transported to satellite kitchens
    b. Food is purchased that needs little to no preparation
    c. Food is produced onsite and then held either heated or chilled, and then served to the consumer
    d. Food is cooked fully, then chilled rapidly and stored at controlled temperatures for up to five days

15. Which of the following are factors affecting bacterial growth?
    a. Keeping food out of the temperature danger zone
    b. Food, acidity, temperature, time, oxygen, and moisture are in proper conditions
    c. Certain bacterium in food produces toxins as they grow and die.
    d. All of the above

16. Which of the following is NOT involved in good personal hygiene?
    a. Washing hands properly
    b. Washing uniform once a week
    c. Avoiding the workplace when ill
    d. Maintaining personal hygiene

17. What system identifies biological, chemical, or physical specific points of potential hazards during the production of food at an operation that can be avoided, prevented, or reduced to safe levels?
    a. Hazard Analysis Critical Control Point System
    b. Hazard Analysis Critical Conservation Plan System
    c. Hazard Analysis Chemical Control System
    d. Hazard Analysis Food Production System

18. Which is true regarding the FDA Food Code?
    a. The code is updated every five years.
    b. States are required to adopt the practices of the *Food Code.*
    c. Each associate of a foodservice operation must receive training on the *Food Code.*
    d. The *Code* acts as a guide for local health departments in creating foodservice programs.

19. Which of the following services is the CDC NOT responsible?
    a. Examining the causes and control of disease
    b. Exploring the outbreaks of foodborne illness
    c. Inspecting foodservice operations bi-annually
    d. Provides educational information for sanitation

20. In what temperatures do microorganisms grow best?
    a. 39°F and 130°F
    b. 45°F and 140°F
    c. 41°F and 135°F
    d. 75°F and 145°F

21. What is the primary role of food additives?
    a. To improve color of food
    b. To lengthen a food product's shelf life
    c. To improve texture of food
    d. To reduce calories in food

22. Which of the following is not one of the three parts to a crisis management plan?
    a. Preparation
    b. Provision
    c. Response
    d. Recovery

23. What three elements should be considered when designing the layout of a kitchen?
    a. Work flow, Contamination, and Equipment accessibility
    b. Square footage, Storage, and Team training
    c. Work flow, Cleanliness, and Staff skills
    d. Menu, Hours of Operation, Service times

24. What company is involved in creating standards for sanitary equipment design and certifies sanitary equipment?
    a. NSF International
    b. Underwriters Laboratories (UL)
    c. Environmental Protection Agency (EPA)
    d. Both A and B

25. Which of the following is a way that operations can reduce post-consumer waste?
    a. Create smaller portion sizes
    b. Offer sides a la carte
    c. Do not offer children's menu
    d. Charge higher price for sharing plates

26. Which practice can a foodservice operation implement to conserve water?
    a. To avoid defrosting, do not freeze meats
    b. Boil pasta at a rapid boil to quicken the process
    c. Get a water audit from water utility
    d. Serve water in smaller glasses

27. Which of the following is not a tactic recommended by the EPA to manage and reduce waste?
    a. Eliminate excessive packaging
    b. Reuse containers when possible
    c. Recycle materials
    d. Wash and reuse plastic utensils

28. Which of the following requires documentation?
    a. Spoilage of a food item
    b. Time and temperature
    c. Stock levels
    d. All of the Above

29. How long is a food allowed to be in the temperature danger zone before it must be thrown away?
    a. Four hours
    b. Three hours
    c. Two hours
    d. It should be thrown away immediately

30. When should an employee's hands be washed?
    a. Only if they are not using gloves
    b. Before food prep
    c. In-between handling different food items
    d. Both B and C

31. Which of the following is a sign or symptom of a foodborne illness?
    a. Vomiting
    b. Miscarriage in women
    c. Double vision
    d. All of the Above

Answer Explanations

1. C: Customer or client satisfaction is crucial in a successful business. Establishments must measure satisfaction to determine the customers' expectations. Various factors are considered. The first factor is sales. Sale trends from month to month and year to year will give insight into high demand seasons, as well as menu items the customers enjoy most. Menu items that do not sell well may be removed from the menu, or the introduction of seasonal items may boost sales during certain times of the year. A second factor in evaluating satisfaction is client feedback. It is important to provide an easily accessible avenue for consumers to provide feedback. Once data is collected, it must be evaluated and then applicable changes, if possible, are implemented. All complaints must be addressed in some manner. More common complaints should be addressed immediately. Other customer concerns may take more planning and thought than a simple solution.

2. A: Product specifications are detailed guidelines and characteristics of products used in a foodservice operation to ensure the correct item is ordered each time and to provide consistency.

3. B: The expected level of quality of the operation must be identified before creating product specifications. The product specifications must reflect the service and atmosphere the restaurant is striving to provide.

4. C: The United States Department of Agriculture (USDA) grades are used for over 300 different food and agricultural items with the goal of providing quality measurements or indicators for consumers. Eggs, poultry, and beef are just a few examples of food products graded by the USDA. The grade determines the quality and value of the product.

5. D: The place of origin of a product indicates exactly where a food item is coming from. This standard is significant due to a number of factors:

- An institution's menu may state that an ingredient is from a certain region
- The flavor and texture of a food may vary from region to region
- Policies may dictate products must not come from a certain region
- Operations may market serving local food to guarantee quality

6. A: The goal of the procurement process is to identify policies and procedures that reflect the operation's concepts and goals. Ordering, receiving, and storing procedures make up the procurement process, as well as clarifying product selection.

7. B: A standardized recipe is one that has been adapted and tested to guarantee it will produce a product consistently each time it is used. Standardized recipes ensure the same food item is produced despite preparation by various people, the yield is predictable, the nutrient profile is accurate, and purchasing food items involves low labor.

8. C: Four acceptable techniques to prevent bacterial growth include:

1. Thaw food in a refrigerator whose temperature is 41°F or below.

2. Submerge food under running drinking water whose temperature is 70°F or lower. The pressure of the running water must remove loose food particles from food. The sink, counter, and other work areas should be sanitized before and after thawing food using this method.

3. If food will be cooked immediately, thaw it in a microwave. This may start the cooking process, so food products must be cooked instantly after thawing.

4. Food can be thawed as part of the cooking process. For example, frozen chicken can go straight in the oven without being thawed. These food products escape the temperature danger zone without bacteria growth.

9. B: To avoid cross-contamination, foods need to be prepared separately. Meat, seafood, and poultry are potential food sources leading to cross-contamination. To limit the risk of food-borne illness, the following procedures should be in place during preparation:

- Work areas, cutting boards, and utensils should be cleaned and sanitized before use. Raw meat should be prepared in a different work area or at a different time than fresh produce.

- Hands should be washed frequently and properly. Foodservice gloves should be changed frequently and before beginning a new task.

- To avoid foods entering the temperature danger zone, only food being prepared should be out of storage.

- Prepared meat should be cooked immediately or returned to the refrigerator until cooking.

10. D: Temperature control safety foods are at high risk for foodborne illness. These foods typically are salads like egg, chicken, tuna, potato, and pasta salads. These salads are initially prepared and typically not cooked, eliminating the opportunity to kill bacteria.

11. D: The as purchased (AP) price is the price of an item when it comes through the door at delivery. Many food items like fresh produce or meat are trimmed, chopped, or cooked during preparation and before serving. The cost of the food item after trimming, chopping, or cooking is the edible portion (EP) price.

12. A: The edible portion (EP) price is the cost of an item after all trimming and assembly is done but before cooking.

13. C: The as served (AS) price is the cost of an item when it is served to the consumer. The AS price is comprised of food costs plus labor costs during preparation.

14. C: Conventional foodservice systems involve food production onsite, then held either heated or chilled, and served to the consumer. Choice *A* describes a commissary system. Choice *B* describes an assembly serve system, and Choice *D* describes a cook-chill system.

15. D: Factors affecting bacterial growth include the following:

- Keeping food out of the temperature danger zone reduces risk of foodborne illness.

- Bacteria can grow rapidly if food, acidity, temperature, time, oxygen, and moisture are in proper conditions for growth.

- Some bacteria may change into a different form, called spores, to protect themselves.

- Certain bacteria produce toxins in food as they grow and die. When humans eat toxins, illness can result. Toxins are not always killed during the cooking process.

16. B: Proper personal hygiene is crucial in the prevention of foodborne illness. Good personal hygiene includes:

- Washing hands frequently and properly
- Washing uniform often
- Maintain personal hygiene
- Upholding good health
- Avoiding the workplace when ill

17. A: A Hazard Analysis Critical Control Point (HACCP) system identifies biological, chemical, or physical hazards at specific points during the production of food at an operation. Identifying these points helps to avoid, prevent, and reduce risks to safe levels.

18. D: The *FDA Food Code* is issued every two years by the FDA and lists the government's recommendations for foodservice regulations with the goal of guiding state health departments to create foodservice inspection programs. However, states are not required to adopt the practices.

19. C: The CDC provides the following services:

- Explores outbreaks of foodborne illness
- Examines the causes and control of disease
- Reports statistical data and case studies in the *Morbidity and Mortality Weekly Report (MMWR)*
- Provides educational information for sanitation
- Conducts an inspection program for cruise ships called the Vessel Sanitation Program

20. C: Microorganisms grow best in temperatures between 41°F and 135°F and subsequently, this range is known as the temperature danger zone. When food is time or temperature abused, it is at a higher risk for foodborne illness. Avoiding the time temperature danger zone is crucial in foodservice.

21. B: Food additives are added to food to lengthen its shelf life. They may also be added to alter food to reduce vulnerability to time and temperature abuse. Examples include nitrates, nitrites, and sulfites.

22. B: Provision is not one of the three parts to a crisis management plan. Despite the training, policies, and procedures put in place, a food-borne illness outbreak or other crisis like power outage, flood, water service interruption, or fire may still occur. Responding to the crisis often dictates the outcome of the scenario. A written crisis management program focuses on three parts: preparation, response, and recovery. These three parts help to streamline the response to a crisis for the best possible outcome.

23. A: The layout design of a kitchen should allow it to be cleaned efficiently. The following elements will be addressed in the design of a kitchen:

- Work flow: the goal of an efficient workflow is to minimize the amount of time food spends in the temperature danger zone, as well as the amount of time food is handled.

- Contamination: a well-designed layout will reduce the risk of cross-contamination.

- Equipment accessibility: having equipment be as accessible as possible will ensure that it will be cleaned regularly.

24. D: Choosing equipment intended for sanitation has been streamlined by organizations like NSF International and Underwriters Laboratories (UL). NSF International composes and issues standards for sanitary equipment design. UL also provides sanitation classification listings for NSF-certified equipment and it also lists products in compliance with their own published environmental and public health (EPH) standards.

25. A: Post-consumer waste is considered waste in a restaurant that occurs after the food is served to the consumer. Post-consumer waste makes up the majority of an operation's waste; however, it is difficult to control. Reducing portion sizes, offering half-portions and children's menus, and ensuring that staff members are properly trained and given the correct portion sizes can reduce an institution's post-consumer waste.

26. C: Employee practices are a crucial area for water sustainability. Integrating effective practices into employee training and company policies will set a standard of the operation's commitment to sustainability. Practices include:

- Defrost meats in refrigerator instead of under running water.
- Keep pasta cookers at a simmer rather than a rapid boil.
- Get a water audit from water utility.
- Practice proper fat, oil, and grease handling best practices.
- Serve water to consumers on request only.

27. D: The Environmental Protection Agency (EPA) recommends three tactics to managing waste:

1. Reduce the amount of waste produced by eliminating excessive packaging.

2. Reuse containers when possible. Chemical containers should never be reused as food containers. Containers must be cleaned and sanitized before reuse.

3. Recycle materials. Recyclables should be stored in a proper place where there is no risk of food or equipment contamination or attracting pests.

Materials that are manufactured to be used only one time should be discarded after the first use.

28. D: Food spoilage, time and temperature of foods and equipment, and stock levels should all be recorded daily to keep records of when temperatures of food were taken, how much food was thrown out due to spoilage, and how much food or product should be ordered. Such records can help an institution identify certain problem areas in the operation.

29. C: Food should not be held at improper temperatures for longer than two hours. If food still remains after two hours, it should be discarded.

30. D: Once an employee's hands are washed, he or she may begin handling food. Single-use gloves should be worn when handling food, and discarded when soiled, beginning a different task, at least every four hours of continued use, and after handling raw meat and before handling ready-to-eat food. Hand washing is a crucial step in food sanitation and should be incorporated into employee training.

31. D: There are multiple signs and symptoms of food-borne illness. The most common are diarrhea, nausea, vomiting, abdominal pain, and fever. Less common symptoms involve bloody diarrhea, double vision, weakness, kidney failure, sepsis, pneumonia, meningitis, and miscarriage in pregnant women.

Management of Food and Nutrition Services

Human Resources

Organizational Structures

<u>Organizational Charts</u>
An organizational chart is a diagram that illustrates how employees fit into the organization. It shows relationship between the various positions and functions within the organization. Solid lines usually depict lines of authority, while dotted lines are used to illustrate staff or advisory positions. The typical organizational chart does not usually show the degree of authority at each level or informal relationships.

<u>Job Descriptions, Specifications, and Classifications</u>
Job descriptions, specifications, and classifications are utilized to outline the skills and types of employees needed within the organization. A job description outlines responsibilities, duties, competencies, and education required to perform a specific job. It matches applicants to a job and is also a tool used during employee evaluations. A job specification is written from a job description and documents the knowledge, skills, education, and experience needed to perform a job. It describes the type of employee that would be ideal for that particular function. Job classifications are most often used in large companies and typically have a pay scale or salary ranges attached to each job classification. It should be an objective description of the responsibilities, tasks, and authority level without consideration of the knowledge, skills, experience level, or education of the employees currently in those roles.

Employment Processes

<u>Procedures for Regulation Compliance</u>
Labor Laws
There are several labor laws in place that companies must abide by when recruiting, hiring, or terminating employment with an individual.

The National Labor Relations Act or Wagner Act was passed in 1935 and guaranteed employees the right to organize and join labor unions. It gave unions the right to become a bargaining agent on behalf of the employees and created the National Labor Relations Board (NLRB). The NLRB responds to claims of unfair labor practices made by employees and is considered to be pro-labor legislation.

The Taft Hartley Labor Act or Labor Management Relations Act was passed 1947 and is considered to be pro-management legislation. It amended the Wagner Act and sought to balance the power between employees and management. It outlined specific unfair union labor practices and outlawed the closed shop. This legislation also made it legal for the government to obtain an injunction against strikes that endanger national health or safety.

The Landrum-Griffin Act or Labor Management Reporting and Disclosure Act was passed in 1959. It created a bill of rights for union members and regulated the internal affairs of unions.

The Civil Rights Act was passed in 1964. It prevents employer discrimination of existing or potential employees on the basis of race, color, or national origin. It is overseen by the Equal Employment Opportunity Commission (EEOC).

The Equal Employment Opportunity Act was passed in 1972. It prevents employer discrimination of existing or potential employees on the basis of race, color, religion, gender, national origin, or political affiliation. Like the Civil Rights Act, it is overseen by the Equal Employment Opportunity Commission (EEOC).

The Fair Labor Standards Act was passed in 1938. It is also referred to as the Minimum Wage Law and was the first legislation to set a minimum wage. It also established that any employee working more than forty hours in one week must be paid overtime pay at a rate of one and a half times their usual hourly wage. This Act was amended in 1963 and is known as the Equal Pay Act and prevents employer discrimination of employees on the basis of gender in payment of wages for equal work.

The Age Discrimination Act of 1967 prevents discrimination of an employee based on age.

The Family Medical Leave Act (FMLA) was passed in 1993 and applies to organizations that employ fifty or more individuals. It provides up to twelve weeks of unpaid leave and prohibits the termination of employment during that time. Employees may take leave for the birth or adoption of a child, care for an immediate family member, or care for themselves if they have a serious medical condition. The employer is required to provide an equal job upon the employee's return, but it does not have to be the same job.

The Americans with Disabilities Act was passed in 1992 and applies to organizations that employ fifteen or more employees. This Act requires that employers provide reasonable accommodations in order for an employee to successfully complete the assigned job duties. Reasonable accommodations include removing barriers, provide wide aisles and doors, installing ramps, providing shelving and phones at an appropriate height, and have flashing alarm lights. Job descriptions must include essential job functions and what is required to fulfill those essential job functions.

The Health Insurance Portability and Accounting Act was passed in 1996 and allows employees to transfer insurance coverage to a new employer's insurance plan and protects health insurance coverage for employees who lose their jobs. It also set standards for electronic medical records and national identifiers for healthcare providers and insurance plans. The Act also contains a Privacy Rule that regulates how protected health information is used and disclosed by health insurers, health care providers, and employer-sponsored health plans.

Union Contracts
The term unionization refers to organizing into a labor union. Workers may form a labor union as a means of collective bargaining with the employer. In collective bargaining, one person represents a group of employees to bargain with the employer. Collective bargaining may be used to negotiate wages, workplace safety, health insurance coverage, or other issues important to employees. There are four main types of unions. In a union shop, all employees must join the union after they have been hired. In an open shop, an employee can decide if they would like to join the union or not. In a closed shop, the employee must be a member of the union before being hired. In an agency shop, all employees must pay the agency fee, but are not required to join. Right to work laws are in place that prevent termination of employment if an employee refuses to join a union if the contract has a union shop clause.

Other laws exist to prevent unions from forcing or putting pressure on employees to join the union. Employers cannot discriminate against employees who refuse to join the union. Laws also prevent an employer from asking an employee about their union activities and cannot refuse to bargain.

Recruitment, Selection, and Orientation

The act of recruitment is locating the best person to fill a job within an organization. Hiring managers may choose to transfer, promote, or rehire an internal candidate to fill a job or seek a new employee from outside the organization. Outside sources include job advertisements, recruiting firms, or unions.

A potential candidate must be interviewed for an open job. Interviews can be structured in such a way that the interviewer asks the same questions of all candidates. This method can reduce personal biases. An unstructured interview has no pre-determined list of questions and the interviewer may ask more open-ended questions. The Fair Employment Practice Law makes it illegal for a potential employer to ask about a candidate's race, religion, gender, national origin, age, or marital status.

Orientation is the process in which an employee learns the skills and behaviors expected in the position, to help them successfully transition into the new organization.

Scheduling

An employee schedule is a time management tool typically used by a supervisor to ensure that an appropriate number of employees are available and are completing all possible tasks, events, or actions needed to meet organizational goals or patient safety standards. It may also be used to keep track of employee hours to help control salary expenses and reduce overtime.

Productivity and Work Simplification

Work Simplification

Work simplification is the thought process in which tasks are performed in the simplest, easiest, and most efficient manner. It focuses on the smallest parts of the job. The goal of work simplification is to reduce inefficiencies by identifying and eliminating unnecessary parts of a job. This helps to increase productivity and decrease expenses. An example of work simplification may include changing the workflow in the kitchen to reduce the number of steps employees walk between stations.

Performance Standards and Competencies

Performance standards are developed by the management of an organization and are documentation of the requirements and expectations of a job. They should be objective, measurable, realistic, and clearly stated. The standards should be used during an annual employee evaluation to measure performance in the employee's current job function.

Competencies are the knowledge, skills, and abilities that an individual must possess in order to be successful in their job. Competency is usually gained through formal education, work experience, and on-the-job training. Measuring employee competency should be a part of annual performance appraisals to ensure that the right people are in the right roles. It should be noted that competence is an employee's capacity to perform the tasks required, while performance is what the employee actually does. Competency can predict performance, although a competent employee may not perform the job effectively. Competency can be measured in several ways, including written tests or chart review, or inferred from work observation.

Performance Appraisals and Documentation

A performance appraisal should be an annual process to assess an employee's job performance in relation to an established job description, specifications, and performance standards. It can be an opportunity to help an employee learn what skills are required for job growth and development. Documentation of performance appraisals should be the same for all employees and would ideally include objective assessments in addition to subjective assessments. Forms should be signed by the employee, the person conducting the performance appraisal, and the employee's immediate manager (if they are not conducting the appraisal) and placed in the employee's permanent file. If the employee fails to meet performance standards, a written plan should be in place on what is expected of the employee and what resources will be available to help the employee meet performance goals.

<u>Personnel Actions</u>
A promotion occurs when an employee is moved to another job that involves a higher wage, increased level of responsibility and performance needs, and usually a higher status within the organization. Management may use promotions as an incentive for improving performance.

A transfer occurs when an employee is moved to another job at generally the same level, the same basic wage, and the same level of responsibility and performance needs. It allows employers to place employees where the need is the greatest or provide employees with jobs they prefer.

A separation may be voluntary (resignation) or involuntary (termination). Involuntary separation must have adequate documentation describing the events leading to the termination.

Compensation is typically broken down into two categories: salary and wages. A salary is a set amount of money provided for a job regardless of the hours worked to perform that job. It is usually designated for managerial and professional employees. Wages are hourly earnings and are subject to the Fair Labor Standards Act. Employees earning an hourly wage may be found at multiple levels within an organization.

Benefits fall into three different categories. Statutory benefits are mandated by law and provide income to an individual in the event of unemployment, injury on the job, or death on the job. Compensatory benefits are earned vacation or paid time off; an employee is paid or receives other benefits for time not worked. Supplementary benefits are usually health insurance and life insurance offered and managed by the employer.

<u>Retention</u>
Employee retention refers to an organization's ability to retain employees. It is gaining more attention as organizational management recognizes the significant costs associated with recruiting, hiring, and training new employees. Organizations may provide flexible work schedules to promote work/life balance, offer unique benefits, or extensive training programs to help improve retention rates.

<u>Diversity</u>
Workplace diversity describes a company's workforce, specifically employee characteristics such as age, gender, ethnicity, work experiences, religion, or sexual orientation. The workplace is becoming increasingly diverse, better reflecting the general population characteristics of the United States.

Finance and Materials

Budget Development

A budget is an estimate of income and expenses for a certain period of time, usually one year. Organization management determines a budget to help estimate future needs and provides a basis for control of expenditures. While budgets are often set for an entire year, they must be reviewed monthly for accuracy and must be flexible to change as the organization's needs change.

<u>Financial Objectives</u>
Financial objectives are set by management and often include specific goals on generating revenue and controlling costs. They should be specific and measured in monetary terms. Financial objectives can help management understand if the company is meeting certain goals that affect overall profitability and long-term viability of the organization.

<u>Budget Types</u>
Operations
An operations or operating budget is commonly defined as a detailed projection of all income and expenses based on sales revenue forecast during a certain period of time. Most organizations write operations budgets for the period of twelve months. The first step in planning an operations budget is to forecast sales or revenue. The second step involves budgeting for expenditures (such as labor or operating expenses) needed for the projected level of revenue.

Capital
A capital budget is used to forecast costs associated with large purchases such as machinery, facility improvements, and long-term service contracts and usually includes expenditures that are expected to last longer than twelve months.

Other
There are several types of budgets and a company may use several at one time. A cash flow budget projects revenues and expenses and how cash will flow into and out of the organization. It can help determine if funds are available when needed. A capital budget is used for items in which the expenditure is expected to last for longer than one year. A zero-based budget begins at zero and is planning oriented. Previous allocations or expenditures are not the basis for future projections. Each expense in a zero-based budget must be justified. A master budget is an aggregate of all of the company's budgets and is often used in large organizations.

Financial Analysis

<u>Labor</u>
Labor is a term often used by the management of an organization to describe the amount of work required to complete specific tasks as outlined in job specifications. Labor costs are usually closely monitored and tracked by management, though it can be difficult to control.

Productivity management is an important evaluation tool to help measure efficiency of the workforce and make decisions regarding staffing and resource allocation. One measure of productivity is to evaluate the number of meals produced per labor hour. To determine the number of meals produced per labor hour, the number of meals produced is divided by the total number of hours worked. For example, if the manager determined that there was a total of 600 labor hours worked during the previous week and there were 900 meals produced during the week:

$$\frac{900 \text{ meals produced}}{600 \text{ hours worked}} = 1.5 \text{ meals produced per labor hour during the previous week}$$

Hiring and training employees is expensive for an organization. Employees may need to be replaced due to retirement, resignations, transfers, or terminations. The labor turnover rate is a ratio that compares the total number of separations to the average monthly employment for a set period of time. For example:

In the past six months, ten employees in the department of eighty employees were replaced. To find the turnover ratio, divide the total number of employees that were separated by the total number of employees in the department and multiply by 100.

$$10/80 \times 100 = 12.5\%$$

Food

Food costs are typically the most easily controlled item in the budget, although it is often subject to greatest amount of fluctuation. Thoughtful menu planning is the most important step in planning for and managing food costs. Flexible menus can help control costs when commodity prices fluctuate. Careful employee training in food preparation and service can help control waste, improve production efficiency, and standardize portions. Participation in group purchasing organizations can lead to improved purchasing power and reduced prices. Proper storage of food and inventory management can help decrease waste due to food spoilage or expiration.

Some equations that can help a manager determine food costs include:

Edible Portion (EP) vs. As Purchased (AP) Prices
The formula below is to find the EP cost of a product.

$$\frac{Raw\ Purchase\ Cost\ (AP)}{Cooked\ Edible\ Weight} = EP\ Cost$$

For example, the purchasing manager purchases twenty pounds of raw ground beef at $1.50 per pound to make a lasagna recipe. The net amount of ground beef available for the recipe after cooking is only eighteen pounds. To determine the cost of the edible portion, divide the purchase cost by the edible weight.

$$Raw\ purchase\ cost\ is\ 20 \times 1.50 = \$30$$

$$Then,\ 30 \div 18\ pounds = \$1.68$$

Therefore, the cost of the edible portion of ground beef is $1.68 per pound

Turnover Ratios
Turnover ratios are a useful management tool to determine how often certain items are consumed and replenished. A turnover rate of two to four times per month is considered to be a desirable level. A low turnover ratio may indicate that large amounts of money are tied up in inventory and can lead to food spoilage. A very high turnover ratio may indicate limited inventory kept on hand, a high amount of waste, employees not following standardized recipes, or theft.

$$\frac{Cost\ of\ Sales\ (food\ cost)}{Average\ Inventory\ Cost}$$

Example: The food cost for the month of December was $65,890 while the average inventory cost was $23,350. To determine the inventory turnover ratio:

$$\$65,890 \div \$23,350 = 2.82$$

Inventory turned over 2.8 times during the month of December.

Food Cost Per Meal

The food cost can be determined by adding all of the food purchases for the month to the cost of foods removed from inventory or by subtracting the value of inventory at the beginning of the month from the value of the inventory at the end of the month and adding all food purchases. To determine the food cost per meal, a manager will need the number of meals served, the total amount of food purchases, and the total amount of food removed from inventory.

$$\frac{\text{Food Cost Per Month}}{\text{Number of Meals Per Month}}$$

Example: It was determined that the total value of inventory as of April 1st was $45,725, and the total value of inventory on May 1st was $39,180. Total food purchases in April totaled $66,345. The total number of meals served in April was counted at 59,000. To determine the food cost per meal:

$$\frac{(45,725 - 39,180) + 66,345}{59,000}$$

Total cost per meal was $1.24 in April.

Capital

The term *capital* generally refers to resources available for use, such as money or equipment. Financial analysis involving capital seeks to determine the financial health of an organization and its sustainability.

The working capital ratio is:

$$\frac{\text{Current Assests}}{\text{Current Liabilities}}$$

It indicates whether or not an organization has enough short-term assets (such as cash and inventory) to cover its short-term debt. Anything less than one indicates a negative working capital and poor financial health of the organization.

The profit margin calculation is the most commonly used assessment of the overall financial picture of an organization. It reflects the portion of sales volume remaining after paying all expenses.

$$\frac{\text{Net profit (cash remaining after paying all expenses)}}{\text{Sales Dollars (revenue)}}$$

Other

Direct costs are costs that are directly associated with the service to the customer. Examples include cost of food, china, silver, uniforms, laundry, employee benefits, or equipment maintenance.

Indirect or fixed costs exist regardless of the sales volume and are required to keep the business open and operating. Examples include rent, taxes, insurance, or asset depreciation. Profit is defined as the income an organization realizes after it pays all of its direct and indirect costs. A loss for the organization occurs when its costs and expenses exceed revenue.

Cost Controls and Materials Management

In a food service organization, cost controls should be in place for purchasing, receiving, storage, issuing, preparation, cooking, and service. Standardized recipes, which include portion size, should be followed each time a dish or menu item is prepared to ensure proper number of portions and cost per portion per batch. Recipe cost cards may be used to calculate what the cost of a standard portion should be for a menu item. Controlling the food cost percentage (the relationship between the dollar amount of sales and the cost of the food in those sales) is one of the cornerstones in a profitable food service operation.

The use of standardized recipes helps to make production more uniform, ensuring consistent quality and an increased efficiency in inventory management. Inventory should be monitored closely to ensure that products are ordered as they are needed, avoiding shortages and preventing products from going to waste.

The FIFO system (first in-first out) of inventory management can help ensure that the oldest products or ingredients are used first, to reduce the risk of expiration or spoilage. Poor inventory management greatly increases costs and reduces profitability.

Standard operating procedures should be in place for product delivery. The organization should establish certain receiving hours and have dedicated individuals responsible for checking in orders to ensure correctness and freshness. Those individuals should be responsible for stocking new inventory following the FIFO system.

The menu is also a critical tool in the profitability of a food service operation. Food costs influence what goes on a menu and it should reflect overall operational costs. In a commercial food service environment, the menu is an important sales tool, and menu prices should include all of the costs associated with buying, preparing, and serving the food in addition to the fixed costs of keeping the facility open. In a non-retail food service environment, the menu offered to patients or residents should promote customer satisfaction, and management should be aware of all of the factors that influence food costs.

Financial Performance Monitoring and Evaluation

Financial statements, such as a balance sheet and a profit/loss statement or income statement, are beneficial in judging a food service operation's viability. The balance sheet illustrates the financial position at a certain point in time, such as at the end of a month, quarter, or year. It specifies assets (cash, inventory, supplies, receivables, building, equipment, etc.), liabilities (depreciation, current payables, long term debt, etc.), and any equity. In short, it demonstrates what the organization owns as well as anything it owes to other companies.

The profit/loss statement or income statement summarizes the organization's sales, costs, and expenses incurred during a certain period of time such as a month, quarter, or year. It provides a snapshot of an organization's ability to generate profit. It may be useful to compare an income statement from different accounting periods to spot changes in sales, costs, or expenses.

Net income is the total profit an organization earns on each dollar of revenue or sales. It is usually expressed as a percentage.

Cash flow is the total amount of money that comes into and out of an organization. Cash flow management is key to paying vendors and employees in a reliable and timely fashion. Problems with cash flow could signal poor inventory control (ordering too often), improper menu pricing, or large amounts of waste (not following standardized recipes), or theft.

Marketing Products and Services

Marketing Principles

Techniques and Methods

Marketing analysis is the process of identifying a need, potential clients, and filling that need. The need identified is a product or service that is offered in exchange for money or something else of value. It is critical to conduct a thorough analysis of potential clients, location, and potential products and services to offer in the marketplace.

The first step in the marketing planning process is to identify a need that is not being filled. This is often referred to as a market niche. The process of dividing the market into groups with similar product needs is the process of market segmentation. A target market is the group of people with similar needs with the potential for purchasing a product or service.

The next step often involves conducting a formal or informal survey of the target market to determine if the need the organization identified matches the need in the marketplace. Healthcare organizations may also glean important information about how to improve a service or introduce a new service from patient satisfaction surveys.

Preparation and Implementation

If the marketing strategy involves offering a new product or service, it is important that all employees receive training on new processes required to offer the new service. New products and services should be introduced to employees well in advance of the marketing campaign launch date so they can be prepared to answer questions and effectively promote the new offering. It is best to keep the marketing plan simple and flexible with clearly defined action steps and a timeline as to when the steps should be accomplished prior to the launch of the new product or service.

Some organizations may decide to have a "test" day and offer a limited number of customers the new product or service to determine if employees have received enough training and gauge what changes may need to be made in the kitchen, cafeteria, or in delivery.

Evaluation

It is important that the marketing strategy has a clear plan about how to reach marketing goals. The marketing strategy should have clearly defined, quantifiable, attainable goals written in the form of objectives and may cover the average number of customers to serve each day or a target number of special catering events during a certain season.

After a selected period of time, sales records, inventory records, cost of food reports, or profit statements are used to analyze if the marketing strategy was a success in terms of the predefined marketing objectives. If the marketing strategy is not meeting objectives, it is important for management to be flexible and modify the strategy to help realize goals.

Marketing Strategies

The 4 Ps of Marketing

There are 4 Ps in marketing: product, place, promotion, and price. The product is a good, service, or an idea. It should fit the need identified during the marketing planning process. The place is where and how the product or service is offered. Promotion is an important part of marketing and used to increase awareness of the product or service offered. Some examples of promotion include local radio or television news releases, direct mail pieces, paid advertisements in the local paper, or running a contest. The use of social media has become an important promotional activity that can help reach the target audience in a cost-effective manner. The price should be set after careful consideration of costs and what the marketplace will accept.

There are several different techniques that are often used to determine pricing:

Factor Method
The factor method is a traditional method in which the mark-up factor is multiplied by the raw food price to determine the final selling price. Ten percent is often added to the food cost to cover losses in cooking and preparation and unproductive costs. Formula:

$$100 \div food\ cost\ percentage = markup\ factor$$

Example: Food cost percentage is 25 and the raw food cost of the menu item is:

$$\$2.75.\ 100 \div 25 = 4\ markup\ factor$$

$$4 \times 2.75 = \$11.00$$

If the 10% hidden cost factor is going to be included, the final selling price will be:

$$4 \times (2.75 + 0.28) = \$12.12$$

Prime Cost Method
The prime cost method is used when raw food costs and direct labor costs are factored into the final selling price of the menu item. The selling price is determined by multiplying the prime cost by the mark-up factor. The mark-up factor is determined by management. Example: The raw food cost of the menu item is $4.19. Total labor time to make the menu item is approximately 12 minutes at a rate of $15 per hour for a total labor cost of $3.00. The food cost percentage was determined to be .333 and the labor cost percentage was determined to be .45.

$$\begin{array}{ll} \text{Raw food cost} & 4.19 \\ \underline{\text{Labor cost}} & \underline{\quad 3.00} \\ \text{Prime Cost} & 7.19 \end{array}$$

To determine the mark-up factor:

Food cost percentage .333 plus labor cost percentage .45 equals 0.783 or 78%.

$$100 \div 78 = 1.28$$

Selling price $= 7.19 \times 1.28 = \$9.20$.

Promotions Pricing
Promotions pricing is utilized during a short period of time to increase sales during a slow period.

Cost of Profit Pricing
Cost of profit pricing is utilized when management is interested in a predetermined percentage of profit on each sale of an item. Profit is established as part of the cost of the item. To determine the price of an item using the profit pricing method, add up all of the costs, including the profit, as a percentage. To find

the targeted food cost percentage, subtract the total of the costs from 100%. Finally, to determine the final selling price of the item, divide the total food cost by the desired food cost percentage.

For example:

Food cost is $1.08
Fixed cost 20%
Labor cost 35%
Profit cost 15%
Total cost 70%
To find the targeted food cost percentage: $100\% - 70\% = 30\%$
To find the selling price $1.08 \div .30$ desired food cost percentage
Selling price = $3.60

Management Principles and Functions

Management serves to plan, organize, direct, and control the direction and the function of the company.

Management Principles

<u>Approaches</u>
Motivational Theories and Strategies
Maslow's Hierarchy of Needs is a motivational theory that provides a personal incentive for the employee. It states that a person's basic needs—such as air, food, water, safety, or security—must be met before an employee can focus on higher needs that can lead to self-actualization, realization of full potential, advanced training, and job enrichment. Examples of the higher human needs include the need to feel accepted, the need for praise, rewards, and promotions. Once the basic needs are met, the higher needs can become motivators for an employee.

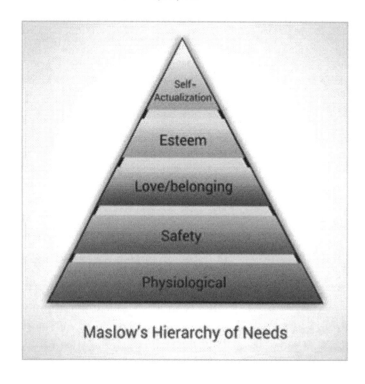

Maslow's Hierarchy of Needs

Herzberg's theory is a motivation and maintenance approach method. The maintenance factors are the wages and the physical conditions in which the employee is asked to work and are not useful in producing motivation. These maintenance factors can be either satisfiers or dis-satisfiers. Dis-satisfiers may interfere with an employee's motivation and keep an employee from reaching his or her full potential. Recognition, responsibility, participation in decision-making, opportunity for growth and advancement, and personal accomplishment are the true motivators that lead to job enrichment and employee enthusiasm.

McClelland's Achievement-Affiliation Theory suggests that all people have the need to achieve, the need for power, and a need for affiliation. People with the desire or need to do something better or more efficiently tend to gravitate towards sales and management positions. They are task-oriented and can be good self-motivators. People with the need for affiliation have the desire to be liked by others. People with the need for power like competitive environments and may seek confrontation.

The MacGregor theory about management asserts that the attitude of the manager toward employees has an impact on job performance. Theory X is inherently negative and states that people dislike work and will avoid it, if possible. Managers who follow this theory believe in an autocratic style of management, controlling and directing employee tasks, using fear for motivation. A manager who follows the Theory Y approach believes that work is a natural activity and that management should provide an environment that is positive and participative. These types of managers believe that employees can achieve company goals and objects by directing their own efforts and do not need to be micromanaged to stay on task.

The Hawthorne Studies were conducted at a textile plant to determine why employee turnover rate was so high and how to decrease it. Elton Mayo was one of the original interpreters of these studies, and he concluded that employees were more productive and more interested in their work when they received special attention by management. In other words, special attention improves behavior and motivation. The phrase "the Hawthorne Effect" was coined by a later interpretation of the studies and describes the increase in employee motivation and productivity as temporary. The differences in employee productivity are a direct result of the employee being aware that he or she is being observed.

The Expectancy theory of motivation states that rewards serve as motivators for employees, but only under certain circumstances. The employees must feel that performance leads to certain rewards and that these rewards must be important for the employee to attain. Employees are more motivated when they feel that a certain level of individual effort will lead to achieving the organization's goals and objectives.

Classical/Traditional Management Approaches
This is a formal structure that organizes and administers all work activities. The main responsibility of management is to coordinate all employees and their activities to ensure company goals and objectives are met. Managers focus on needed tasks, promoting authority, and enforcing structure. An organizational chart in this type of company would illustrate that each employee is only accountable to one supervisor or manager and that the chain of command flows in a direct line from the highest levels of management down to the first level of the company. This type of structure often receives the criticism that it does not allow for group interactions and cross-collaboration in the decision-making process.

Behavioral Management Approaches
This type of structure follows a participative approach to leadership and uses behavioral sciences as a cornerstone to form organizational and management structure. Theory Z, sometimes used in companies that follow human relations management styles, states that employees are extremely valuable to the organization and believes in a consensus decision-making process. Managers feel that allowing employees to participate in the decision-making process improves morale and productivity.

Integration Management Approaches
This type of structure lends itself to an open and interactive environment in a company. Managers who follow this type of approach believe that the company is made up of many interdependent parts and that changes in one part of the company will influence other parts of the company. Managers should look outside of their immediate department when making big decisions. Managers must use information from other departments that may have conflicting goals and objectives and incorporate that into the decision-making process for their own departments.

Skills
Technical skills, the understanding of and proficiency in a specific kind of task or activity, are the most important at lower levels of management.

Human skills, the ability to work effectively as part of a group, are important at all levels of an organization, but are critical in lower levels of management.

Conceptual skills are the ability to see the organization as a whole, and the importance of this skill increases at higher levels of management.

Roles
Information Giving
There are three types of informational roles: monitor, disseminator, and spokesman. The manager in a monitor role is one who is constantly searching for information. The disseminator provides information to the employees in his or her department while the spokesman communicates information to people both inside and outside of the organization.

Conflict Resolution
Conflict within a department or an organization as a whole is inevitable and sometimes can lead to very positive changes. A good manager does not suppress or resolve all conflict, but instead manages the conflict and attempts to control any harmful aspects and maximize beneficial aspects of the conflict. There are three main methods utilized when attempting to resolve conflict within an organization. A dominance and suppression method suppresses conflict and creates an environment where one party feels like the winner while the other feels like the loser. A forceful manager may attempt to force his or her position upon another employee while a smoothing manager may try to minimize the conflict by influencing one employee to agree with another. Neither of these methods actually resolves the conflict. A manager may simply avoid the conflict by refusing to take a position, postponing action, or acting as if he or she is unaware of the issue. Conflict may be resolved by majority vote. This could be effective as long as all employees involved feel that the procedure is fair and presents a balanced perspective.

Compromise can be a successful approach to conflict resolution by finding middle ground between employees involved in the dispute. Compromise is the most effective when each side feels that they are asked to sacrifice equally while still achieving some of their goals. The solution that is reached may be such that all employees involved feel satisfied with the outcome but may not ultimately solve the conflict.

Problem Solving

Integrative problem solving is a hands-on approach to conflict resolution in which involved employees openly and jointly try to find a solution that is acceptable to all. When well managed, this can be an effective tool to solve conflict and find solutions that can help make the organization stronger.

Decision-Making

Decision-making and problem solving are important skills for all employees of an organization, regardless of their level. The decision-making process involves the following steps: recognize and analyze the problem, determine workable solutions, gather data, select plausible solutions, take action on the solutions, and follow-up on the actions.

The Delbecq technique for decision-making is a very structured and controlled brainstorming group with an authoritative leader, clearly focused goals, clearly defined procedures, and controlled interactions between group members. Ideas provided by group members are recorded and ranked by the group. The group votes on the ideas and uses the majority vote as the final decision.

The Delphi technique to decision-making utilizes experts in a series of interviews from which a consensus decision can be made. The participants normally do not meet in person and are usually from outside of the organization.

A fish diagram creates an illustration of a particular problem or situation. It focuses on different causes of a problem and categorizes internal and external factors related to the problem. The diagram is a series of connected arrows with each arrow representing a different factor related to the problem. This technique increases employee involvement in decision-making and asks group participants to think about the causes and effects of the current situation.

Communication

Clear communication is critical at all levels of an organization. Communication at the organizational level can be conducted in downward, upward, horizontal, or diagonal channels. A downward communication channel is one in which communications come from the department manager and flow down to the employees. Upward communication channels carry communications from the employees up to department managers. Horizontal communication channels flow between different departments at the same level in the organization. Diagonal communication channels serve to help communication happen more quickly. An example may be an employee sending an order request directly to the purchasing department rather than sending the order request to his or her department manager first.

Managers must have good listening skills as a part of good interpersonal communication skills. They should be hands on and clearly explain the purpose behind company policies, procedures, and expectations.

Planning

Short and Long Range

Short range or operational planning typically covers one year and often coincides with the operating budget. Long range planning covers up to a five-year plan and requires a mission statement to help ensure objectives are met.

Strategic and Operational

Strategic planning focuses on high-level decisions for the direction of the company rather than on specific plans and objectives. Part of strategic planning includes conducting a SWOT analysis. SWOT is an acronym for strengths, weaknesses, opportunities, and threats and is a useful tool that can assist management in identifying internal and external forces that can impact the company. When done correctly, SWOT analysis can reveal both positive forces and possible problems that need to be addressed. Strengths can be internal or external qualities that help the organization meet goals and objectives. Weaknesses should be analyzed from both an internal and external perspective and can keep the organization from meeting goals and objectives. Opportunities take place in the external environment and are often things that are out of control of management. Threats are conditions external to the company that can threaten the overall stability and sustainability of the company. SWOT analyses can be very subjective, based on the opinions and experience of the individuals conducting the analysis. It requires a great deal of research and knowledge of the company, industry, regulatory environment, and competitors, among others. Incomplete research can lead to a weak SWOT analysis that ultimately may not prove to be beneficial in the strategic planning of the company.

<u>Policies and Procedures</u>
Planning is the basic function of management. Predetermined objectives guide management's decisions. Management sets policies that outline parameters on acceptable and expected behaviors and activities. Procedures outline expectations on daily operations and tasks.

<u>Disaster Preparedness</u>
Disaster preparedness is critically important, especially in regions that may be susceptible to natural disasters. Plans should be written down and regularly reviewed and practiced with staff. Disaster preparedness should be incorporated into new employee orientation. Emergency evacuation plans or where to take shelter should be posted in obvious locations. Management should maintain current and accurate records of employee names, addresses, phone numbers, and emergency contact numbers. Phone numbers for OSHA, HAZMAT, Poison control, and who within the organization to contact in the event of an emergency should be posted. Employees should be informed of where to find menus and recipes in the event a regular menu cannot be followed, due to limited power or water supplies.

During emergency situations, employees must continue to follow safe food practices. Temperatures of refrigeration and freezer units should be monitored closely in the event of limited power. Authorized personnel should prepare and serve food. Paper products should be utilized if limited power or water will prevent a dishwasher from reaching proper temperatures for cleaning and sanitizing.

Organizing

<u>Structure/Design of Department/Unit</u>
The organization of the department or a unit serves to identify the tasks and activities that must be accomplished and divides those tasks into different positions. The organizational structure also helps to establish relationships between all positions within the same department and other departments and management of the company.

A company with a narrow span of control requires more managerial levels and often requires more managers. In contrast, a company with a wide span of control has fewer managerial levels and is effective when employing highly trained and highly motivated workers.

Staff may function in a variety of ways within a department or unit:

- Advisory staff is not involved with the day-to-day operations of the department or unit and have supportive roles. For example, a consultant dietitian may be hired for menu planning and meal analysis to support nutritional goals but is not involved in the purchasing, preparation, or delivery of meals.

- Functional staff often have specialized knowledge in a particular area of the department but often haven limited authority. They may help line workers when needed with specific tasks or may act in an advisory manner.

- Other staff may be referred to as line workers or kitchen staff. These employees are responsible for all tasks related to the preparation and cleanup of meals. They should be well trained in proper food handling and cooking techniques to prevent food borne illness and employee injury. Cross training is an effective tool to help reduce disruptions in service when line workers are out.

In the acute care setting, most managers use an index of seventeen minutes per meal or 3.5 meals per labor hour to determine staffing needs. Extended care facilities often use an index of five meals per labor hour, while a cafeteria manager may use an index of 5.5 meals per labor hour. School foodservice cafeteria managers often use an index between thirteen and fifteen meals per labor hour when determining staffing needs. The work schedule should be based on an eight-hour day with one thirty-minute meal break and one or two fifteen-minute breaks.

Establishing Priorities

Establishing priorities is an important aspect of a properly functioning foodservice system. Staff should be trained on which tasks should take priority over others and why this is the case. Time management is a useful tool and skill that should be utilized by foodservice workers in order to ensure that all tasks are completed in a timely manner. For example, food items that require more time to prepare should be given priority over others. Also, food safety techniques should always be given top priority.

Tasks/Activities and Action Plans

A work schedule can be a useful tool to help prioritize tasks and activities. The master schedule serves as the overall plan for how employee time is to be used and also tracks any vacations and days off and on. The master schedule should serve as the basis for developing weekly work schedules. A shift schedule has a narrow focus and tracks the number of hours and days worked per week. A production schedule informs employees of their specific assignments and what tasks need to be accomplished and when. It can be organized on a daily and weekly basis depending on the number of tasks to be accomplished and management preference.

Resource Allocation

Resource allocation is a process of assigning resources, such as employees or equipment, to various tasks. Resources should be allocated in a manner that considers efficiency, cost effectiveness, and individual employee skills. A food production chart which approximates the amount of productive and nonproductive time in food preparation can be helpful when assigning resources and planning production.

Food costs are the most readily controlled item in a budget and in menu planning but are subject to the greatest fluctuation. Menu planning is a critical step in controlling food costs. Limiting menu items can help reduce waste and control costs. Storage control (inventory management), production control (standardized recipes), and standardized portions are also important parts of controlling food costs. If meals are offered to employees, department management should keep accurate records of food given to employees and separate the cost of those meals from meals sold or given to patients or residents.

Labor costs are not as easily controlled as food costs. Good use of food production charts and employee schedules can help ensure that the food service department is properly staffed, reducing the need for regular overtime and reducing the likelihood of staffing shortages.

Other factors to consider when assigning resources include food safety, patient or resident preferences, availability of skilled employees, patient or resident census, and profitability of any retail sales. Consideration of energy use, water use, food waste, and other environmental factors may become more important factors in the future as managers determine how to assign resources in food service.

Professional Standards of Practice and Development

Roles/Levels of Dietetic Personnel
As outlined by the Academy Quality Management Committee and Scope of Practice Subcommittee of the Quality Management Committee of the Academy of Nutrition and Dietetic, Registered Dietitians (RDs) can work in research, public health settings, healthcare, industry or business, government or military, or in school nutrition ranging from elementary schools to colleges and universities. The Academy of Nutrition and Dietetic encourage RDs to provide culturally competent, individually tailored, safe nutrition messages that enhance the nation's health while advancing the dietetic profession. The RD designation is recognized nationally and is a legally protected title. In order to obtain the RD credential, an individual must complete at least a Bachelor's degree at a U.S. regionally accredited college or university.

In addition to classes in specific food and nutrition sciences, course work also includes psychology, anatomy and physiology, biochemistry, organic chemistry, foodservice systems management, microbiology, and possible genetics. Supervised practice is also required and must be completed through a Didactic Program in Dietetic and Dietetic Internship or a Coordinated Program in Dietetic. Only after all of the course work and supervised practice is completed can an individual sit for the Registration Examination for Dietitians, which is administered by the Commission on Dietetic Registration. A RD must complete 75 hours of continuing professional education credits every five years in order to maintain their RD credential.

In order to obtain a Dietetic Technician, Registered (DTR) credential, an individual must successfully complete at least an Associate's degree at a U.S. regional college or university and a Dietetic Technician Program. The supervised practice program must allow for a minimum of 450 practice hours and must be accredited by the Accreditation Council for Education in Nutrition and Dietetic of the Academy of Nutrition and Dietetic. An individual may also complete a Bachelor's degree in a Didactic Program in Dietetic. Once course work is completed, the individual may sit for the Registration Examination for Dietetic Technicians. Fifty hours of continuing professional education credits are required every five years to maintain the DTR credential.

The RD and DTR may work together in an acute care health care setting during the nutrition care process. The DTR may assist with a nutrition assessment, implement or oversee the interventions as outlined by the RD, and observe and report results of nutrition intervention based on specific monitoring activities assigned by the RD or outlined by institution protocol.

A nationally and legally accepted definition of the term "nutritionist" does not exist. Some states recognize this term and have enacted legislation that regulates the use of the term and outlines specific qualifications required to hold and use this title. However, this varies from state to state. The Academy of Nutrition and Dietetic believes that all RDs are nutritionists but not all nutritionists are RDs.

<u>Legislative Process</u>

In the United States, new laws must originate in the House of Representatives. Bills (written ideas for new laws) are introduced in the House and assigned to one of the twenty-two standing committees. The Chairman of the standing committee or subcommittee to which a bill is assigned determines which bills are going to be considered during that session of Congress. If a bill does not move forward out of the committee, it "dies," and must be reintroduced during the next session of Congress. If the bill does not die in committee, a subcommittee will hold public hearings to gather testimony from people with interest in the bill and those deemed to be experts in that subject matter. The subcommittee and the full committee may hold a markup session to offer amendments to the bill. Once the hearings and markup sessions are held, the committee must vote to kill the bill or vote it out of the committee.

If the bill makes it out of the committee, it goes to the full House for consideration. The Rules Committee then decides how much time to devote to the bill for a debate on the floor and if any of the amendments will be offered. Most bills require only half of the members present to vote in favor for it, in order for it to pass.

In the Senate, a new bill is assigned to one of the sixteen standing committees. A committee may decide to study and amend a bill and release it to the full Senate or to table the bill. Once the bill is released to the Senate floor, the Majority Leader determines which bills will be considered and in the order in which they will be debated. The Majority Leader and the Minority Leader determine how many Senators need to be present for the bill to pass (half or three-fifths).

A bill that has been passed by the House and the Senate moves to a conference committee, which is made up of members from both houses of Congress. This committee reconciles the House version and the Senate version of the bill and is sent back to both houses for final approval. A bill must pass both the Senate and the Congress in identical form before it can be sent to the President.

Once the President has the bill, the bill may be vetoed and sent back to Congress for further debate or signed into law and directed to the appropriate agencies for implementation. The President has ten days to sign or veto a bill.

The Academy of Nutrition and Dietetic is actively involved in legislation and public policy through a number of committees and member groups within the organization. The Academy has identified the following areas as priorities in legislation and public policy development: disease prevention and treatment, nutrition in the lifecycle, food systems and access to food, and quality healthcare.

Quality Processes and Research

Regulatory Guidelines

Healthcare regulation in the United States is complex and is not uniform across the country. It involves local, state, federal, and private organizations in the management of all aspects of the healthcare system.

<u>Federal</u>

Healthcare providers and facilities interact with a variety of regulatory agencies at the federal, state, and local levels to promote safety and quality. A few federal regulatory agencies include the Centers for Disease Control and Prevention (CDC), Centers for Medicare and Medicaid Services (CMS), and the Food and Drug Administration (FDA).

The CDC seeks to prepare healthcare providers for outbreaks of disease and provide education on how to prevent the spread of disease.

The FDA is the regulatory agency that is responsible for issuing alters related to medical errors and negative reactions to medications and treatments. The agency specifically provides oversight of blood products, medical devices, vaccines, biologics, and medications.

The Centers for Medicare and Medicaid (CMS) oversee many of the regulations related to healthcare systems. Government-subsidized medical care coverage is offered through a variety of CMS programs including Medicare, Medicaid, and State Children's Health Insurance Program. CMS is also responsible for ensuring HIPPA compliance. It determines reimbursement for healthcare services and seeks to establish quality standards for cost effective care.

The Agency for Healthcare Research and Quality conducts research aimed at improving the quality of healthcare, cost reduction, improved patient safety, and lowering the rate of medical errors.

State and Local
Healthcare regulations vary from state to state. The extent of regulatory power of state and local agencies over acute care medical facilities, extended care or rehabilitation facilities, assisted living facilities, etc. depends on the laws in that state. Certain laws, such as one that specifies the minimum hospital stays for new mothers or mastectomy patients, are set at the state level. Some states require insurance coverage for specialty formulas, diabetes treatment and supplies, or screenings for cervical or prostate cancer while others do not. Laws that regulate insurance coverage are often set at the state level.

State health departments may work with other state agencies to enforce health professional licensure laws and the regulation and inspection of health care facilities. State and local health departments perform vaccine order management and distribution for all childhood immunizations and a large percentage of adult immunizations.

Private organizations (such as the Commission on Dietetic Registration) are also involved at the state and local levels to administer exams granting professional licenses, certifying specialists, or accrediting dietetic programs. Examples of state or local regulatory agencies include the state or local health departments or specific state agencies aimed at research and quality improvement programs.

Accrediting Agencies
The Joint Commission sets the expectation that quality care will lead to improved outcomes. It is a nonprofit organization that accredits more than 21,000 health care organizations and programs in the United States. Many states recognize accreditation by the Joint Commission as a condition of licensure and the receipt of Medicaid reimbursement. The Joint Commission survey is often done jointly with state authorities and has been instrumental in focusing attention on the importance of patient safety through National Patient Safety Goals.

Quality Process and Implementation

Plans
Effective leadership from management and continuous performance improvement are critical for maintaining quality. Total Quality Management (TQM) is the continuous improvement of organizational processes with the goal of attaining the highest level of quality standards for products and services. There are three elements of TQM: customers, culture, and counting. The customers are the true judges

of quality, and it is vital to seek their feedback and input. The company must establish a culture that establishes quality as a top priority. Counting refers to the measurement of what is considered a high-quality product or service and what needs improvement.

TQM professionals may implement a problem-solving technique known as the PCDA cycle: plan, do, check, act. This technique allows management to stay focused on the plan of what is to be done, how to do it, when to check the results, and how to act on the positive and negative results and if needed, return to the first step to develop another plan.

Continuous Quality Improvement (CQI) is a part of TQM that emphasizes the organization and system rather than specific individuals. It is based on the idea that systems and performance can always improve. Outcome assessments are used to determine if CQI initiatives are successful.

Standards/Criteria/Indicators
In the healthcare setting, the criteria or standards are professionally developed statements that describe the desired outcome of a process or procedure. Determining whether the outcomes are positive or negative may be based on specific medical data such as anthropometrics, biochemical labs, or patient survey results. Documentation must include a timeframe and the sequence of activities and procedures used. Criteria should be relevant, understandable, measurable, behavioral, and achievable.

Indicators are measurement tools that monitor and evaluate important aspects of patient care and management functions. They can serve to direct attention to specific issues within the organization or with specific quality improvement initiatives. Indicators should not be used to direct measures of quality, but rather to describe outcomes, events, or complications of activities.

A rate-based indicator describes the best possible care. For example, 90% of patients admitted with a high risk of malnutrition will be screened within 24 hours of admission.

A sentinel event indicator is a serious event leading to serious physical or psychological injury or death that requires investigation each time it occurs. A sentinel event is always undesirable but is usually avoidable. They are usually written as 0% or 100% (never or always). For example, there will be 0% cases of hospital generated food-borne illness. Another example: 100% of patients with a length of stay of seven days will be screened, regardless of admission diagnosis.

Documentation of Data Collection and Outcomes
Medical organizations often contract with a third-party company to conduct patient surveys to gauge patient satisfaction with their care. Surveys that are mailed to a patient's home or done via an automated phone system are often the most effective means of gathering this information. The use of electronic medical records has made it easier to track and record outcomes based on certain parameters or quality initiatives.

Corrective Actions
Corrective actions are needed when quality criteria or standards have not been met or if a sentinel event has occurred. A corrective action should clearly state the problem or situation and identify the steps needed to effectively address and correct the problem or situation. The steps needed in the corrective action should be as specific to the situation or problem as possible and follow organizational policies and procedures. It is important for the plan to be flexible and accurate. The number of steps and length of the corrective action process depends on the problem or situation, the number of employees involved, and if any customers were affected. Each step should identify the person or persons responsible for task completion, completion due date, and parameters to measure progress.

The FDA published the Code of Federal Regulation Title 21 Part 820—Corrective and Preventive Action that outlines seven steps organizations should follow when developing and implementing corrective actions plans. The seven steps are: analyze data, investigate the cause, identify the necessary action(s) to take, validate effectiveness, implement and record changes, share related information to those involved, and submit for management review.

The HAACP plan, Hazard Control and Critical Care Point, is also a useful tool to review when implementing a corrective action that involves the food service department. This plan tries to prevent problems from occurring in the first place.

Evaluate Effectiveness

When evaluating the effectiveness of a new process, procedure, or standard, it is important to determine if there were any unintended consequences within the affected departments or with customers. It is also important to note if the new standards or procedures triggered any nonconformance from employees and determine why employees were not able to follow the new process, procedure, or standard. Managers need to ensure that all employees are properly informed and trained.

When implementing a corrective action plan, the same questions should be asked and the action plan should be tracked throughout its progression. Data should be reviewed after the corrective action plan is implemented to discover if the plan worked as intended, if similar problems or situations still exist, or if the action plan created any potential new problems.

Report

Reporting and documenting changes are critical in any new process implementation or corrective action plan. Sources of data could be the electronic medical record, food service production logs, temperature logs from freezers, and patient satisfaction survey results, among others. Data should be summarized in a report that clearly outlines why the new process, procedure, standard, or corrective action was needed and the outcomes. Digital photography can also be a useful tool in documentation. Company policies should be followed to ensure that all necessary members of management receive a copy of the report and that it is stored where it can be easily accessed, in case it needs to be reviewed by a regulatory agency.

Research

Identifying Problems

It is important to identify any areas within the organization that are not meeting quality standards, failing to comply with federal or state regulatory agencies, or could trigger a negative outcome for a patient. Triggers that may promote identification of problems could be a change in organizational management, a sentinel event, dropping patient satisfaction scores, or employee noncompliance with policies, among others.

Problems within a healthcare organization could be related to quality improvement, staffing issues, the need for new technology, patient outcomes, employee turnover, food quality, and financial performance of the entire hospital or certain departments or outpatient clinics, among others. Problems that are identified should be prioritized and addressed in a systematic manner. Problems that may compromise patient safety or employee safety should be addressed first. Management must be prepared to fully address any problems identified and must follow through with any corrective actions.

<u>Data Collection</u>
After a problem is identified, data may be collected from the electronic medical record, production logs, temperature logs, food cost reports, sales reports, payroll reports, patient satisfaction surveys, critical incidence reports, financial statements, and the Joint Commission report, among others.

All HIPAA guidelines must be followed if using any patient data, and those researching the problem must only access patient information needed for the research. Data should be securely stored and not be saved directly on any laptop computers, flash drives, or mobile devices.

<u>Reporting</u>
Reporting should follow the standards set by state and/or federal agencies and organizational management. The Agency for Healthcare Research and Quality has developed several formats that may be used in acute care hospitals, as it is their responsibility to collect, analyze, and report data in a standardized manner.

The generic common format allows for the standardized collection of basic information. It includes the following information: type of event, circumstances of the event, patient information, and, reporting/reporter/report information.

Practice Questions

1. Carol worked fifty hours last week and was not paid any overtime. What labor law was violated?
    a. The Equal Opportunity Act
    b. The Fair Labor Standards Act
    c. The Equal Pay Act
    d. The Civil Rights Act

2. Judy and Ben were hired at the same company, and both are employed as line workers in the kitchen. About one month after starting, Judy discovers that Ben is getting paid a higher wage. What labor law has been violated?
    a. The Equal Opportunity Act
    b. The Fair Labor Standards Act
    c. The Equal Pay Act
    d. The Civil Rights Act

3. The manager of the food service department is trying to determine the labor turnover rate. In the past six months, ten employees in the department of eighty employees were replaced. What is the turnover rate?
    a. 12.5%
    b. 15%
    c. 17.5%
    d. 20%

4. The cost of food for the past week was $430 while revenue generated from food sales was $800. What is the food cost percentage?
    a. 24%
    b. 44%
    c. 54%
    d. 64%

5. Which of the following is a paid employee who represents union workers?
    a. The shop steward
    b. The mediator
    c. The arbitrator
    d. The hiring manager

6. An employee wishes to join a union. Legally, the employer is allowed to do which of the following?
    a. Fire the employee.
    b. Attempt to dissuade the employee from joining.
    c. Tell other employees this employee wants to join.
    d. Inform the employee about union dues.

7. The purpose of the organizational chart is to do what?
    a. Illustrate the relationship of the various positions and functions within the organization
    b. Illustrate what tasks each department is expected to perform
    c. Illustrate company goals
    d. Illustrate how the company generates revenue

8. A manager wants to place an ad in the local paper for food service workers. The manager should reference which document to write the ad?
   a. Job specification
   b. Job description
   c. Job classification
   d. None of the above

9. During an interview, the manager asks if the candidate is married. This question violates what law?
   a. The Fair Labor Standards Act
   b. The Equal Employment Opportunity Act
   c. The Fair Employment Practice Law
   d. The National Labor Relations Act

10. _____ is/are the knowledge, skills, and abilities that an individual must possess in order to be successful in their job.
   a. Performance
   b. Competency
   c. Standards
   d. Specifications

11. _____ is what the employee does and can be observed.
   a. Performance
   b. Competency
   c. Standards
   d. Specifications

12. Wages are subject to which law?
   a. Equal Employment Opportunity Act
   b. Taft-Wagner Act
   c. Fair Labor Standards Act
   d. Fair Employment Practice Law

13. Which budget is usually set for a twelve-month period and is based on sales revenue forecast?
   a. Zero based budget
   b. Cash flow budget
   c. Capital budget
   d. Operations budget

14. The manager determined that there was a total of 500 labor hours worked during the previous week, and there were 900 meals produced during the week. How many meals were produced per labor hour?
   a. 2
   b. 1.5
   c. 1.8
   d. 2.1

15. A five-pound whole chicken was purchased for $0.99 per pound. The edible portion of the chicken is 75%. What is the EP cost of the chicken?
   a. $1.32/pound
   b. $1.42/pound
   c. $1.02/pound
   d. $1.52/pound

16. The food cost for the month of December was $65,890 while the average inventory cost was $23,350. The inventory turnover ratio for December was what?
   a. 2
   b. 2.5
   c. 2.8
   d. 3

17. Using the factor method, determine what a menu item should be priced at with a 33% food cost, raw food cost of $1.45, and a labor cost of $5.80.
   a. $4.40
   b. $4.00
   c. $2.90
   d. $10.20

18. Using the prime cost method, determine what a menu item should be priced at with a 33% mark-up factor, a raw food cost of $1.45, a labor cost of $5.80, and a labor factor of 45%.
   a. $4.40
   b. $6.95
   c. $8.50
   d. $9.28

19. According to _____, once the basic needs of the employee are met, the higher needs can become motivators for an employee.
   a. Maslow's Hierarchy of Needs
   b. Herzberg's Theory
   c. Theory X/Theory Y
   d. The Hawthorne Theory

20. What skills are most important at lower levels of management?
   a. Technical
   b. Human
   c. Conceptual
   d. None of the above

21. What skills become more important as an employee achieves higher levels of management?
   a. Technical
   b. Human
   c. Conceptual
   d. None of the above

22. What is the decision-making technique that utilizes participants from outside of the organization.
    a. Delbecq technique
    b. Delphi technique
    c. Fish Diagram technique
    d. Integrative technique

23. What does SWOT stand for?
    a. Strengths, weaknesses, opportunities, testing
    b. Structural, weaknesses, occurrences, threats
    c. Strengths, weaknesses, opportunities, threats
    d. Sustainability, weaknesses, opportunities, threats

24. The manager discovers that an employee did not wash fresh vegetables before chopping them and placing them on the salad bar. The manager should write and implement which of the following?
    a. A corrective action
    b. A disciplinary action
    c. A revised HAACP plan
    d. A critical incident report

25. The nutrition department of the hospital would like to make comments about an upcoming bill. When is the best time to do this?
    a. When the bill is in debate in the Senate
    b. When the bill is in debate in the House
    c. When the bill is in public hearings
    d. When the bill is in committee

26. Which of the following is a part of TQM that emphasizes the organization and systems rather than specific individuals?
    a. Continuous Quality Enhancement
    b. Continuous Quality Improvement
    c. Key Performance Indicators
    d. Key Quality Indicators

27. This type of indicator is a serious event that must be investigated each time it occurs.
    a. Rate based indicator
    b. Critical Occurrence
    c. Sentinel Event
    d. Critical Event

28. The manager decides to use the organization's social media page to advertise a month of special menus in the cafeteria. What part of the marketing mix is the manager using?
    a. Place
    b. Price
    c. Promotion
    d. Product

Answer Explanations

1. B: The Fair Labor Standards Act was passed in 1938. It is also referred to as the Minimum Wage Law and was the first legislation to set a minimum wage. It also established that any employee working more than forty hours in one week must be paid overtime pay at a rate of one and a half times usual hourly wage.

2. C: The Fair Labor Standards Act was passed in 1938. It is also referred to as the Minimum Wage Law and was the first legislation to set a minimum wage. It also established that any employee working more than forty hours in one week must be paid overtime pay at a rate of one and a half times usual hourly wage. This Act was amended in 1963 and is known as the Equal Pay Act and prevents employer discrimination of employees on the basis of gender in payment of wages for equal work.

3. A: To find the turnover ratio, divide the total number of employees that were separated by the total number of employees in the department and multiply by 100. $10 \div 80 \times 100$

4. C: To find the food cost percentage, divide the total amount of revenue generated by the sales of the food by the total cost of the food and multiply by 100. $430 \div 800 \times 100$

5. A: The shop steward is a paid employee that represents union workers.

6. D: Laws exist to prevent unions from forcing or putting pressure on employees to join the union. They cannot discriminate against employees who refuse to join the union. Laws also prevent an employer from asking an employee about their union activities and cannot refuse to bargain.

7. A: An organizational chart is a diagram that illustrates how employees fit into the organization. It shows the relationship of the various positions and functions within the organization. Solid lines usually depict lines of authority while dotted lines are used to illustrate staff or advisory positions. The typical organizational chart does not usually show the degree of authority at each level or informal relationships.

8. B: A job description documents responsibilities, duties, competencies, and education required to perform a specific job.

9. C: The Fair Employment Practice Law makes it illegal for a potential employer to ask about a candidate's race, religion, gender, national origin, age, or marital status.

10. B: Competencies are the knowledge, skills, and abilities that an individual must possess in order to be successful in their job. Competency is usually gained through formal education, work experience, and on-the-job training.

11. A: It should be noted that, competence is an employee's capacity to perform the tasks required while performance is what the employee actually does.

12. C: Wages are subject to the Fair Labor Standards Act, passed in 1938.

13. D: An operations or operating budget is commonly defined as a detailed projection of all income and expenses based on sales revenue forecast during a certain period of time. Most organizations write operations budgets for the period of twelve months. The first step in planning an operations budget is to forecast sales or revenue.

14. C: To determine the number of meals produced per labor hour, divide the number of meals produced by the total number of hours worked.

15. A: $1.32/pound. To determine the edible portion cost, divide the raw purchase cost by the cooked edible weight.

16. C: 2.8. To determine the inventory turnover ratio, divide the food cost by the average inventory cost.

17. A: $4.40. The factor method is a traditional pricing method in which the mark-up factor is multiplied by the raw food price to determine the final selling price. Ten percent is often added to the food cost to cover losses in cooking and preparation and unproductive costs.

18. D: $9.28. The prime cost method is used when raw food costs and direct labor costs are factored into the final selling price of the menu item. The selling price is determined by multiplying the prime cost by the mark-up factor. The mark-up factor is determined by management.

19. A: Maslow's Hierarchy of Needs is a motivational theory that provides a personal incentive for the employee. It states that a person's basic needs (examples include air, food, water, safety, security, fair wage, or an acceptable schedule) must be met before an employee can focus on higher needs that can lead to self-actualization, realization of full potential, advanced training, and job enrichment. Examples of the higher human needs include the need to feel accepted, the need for praise, rewards, and promotions. Once the basic needs are met, the higher needs can become motivators for an employee.

20. A: Technical skills are the most important at lower levels of management. It is the understanding of and proficiency in a specific kind of task or activity.

21. C: Conceptual skills are the ability to see the organization as a whole, and the importance of this skill increases at higher levels of management.

22. B: The Delphi technique to decision-making utilizes experts in a series of interviews from which a consensus decision can be made. The participants normally do not meet in person and are usually from outside of the organization.

23. C: SWOT stands for Strengths, Weaknesses, Opportunities, Threats.

24. A: Corrective actions are needed when quality criteria or standards have not been met or if a sentinel event has occurred. A corrective action should clearly state the problem or situation and identify the steps needed to effectively address and correct the problem or situation. The steps needed in the corrective action should be as specific to the situation or problem as possible and follow organizational policies and procedures. It is important for the plan to be flexible and accurate. The number of steps and length of the corrective action process depends on the problem or situation, the number of employees involved, and if any customers were affected. Each step should identify the person or persons responsible for task completion, completion due date, and parameters to measure progress.

25. C: If a bill does not die in a House committee, a subcommittee will hold public hearings to gather testimony from people with interest in the bill and those deemed to be experts in that subject matter.

26. B: Continuous Quality Improvement is a part of TQM that emphasizes the organization and systems rather than specific individuals.

27. C: A sentinel event is a serious event that must be investigated each time it occurs.

28. C: Promotion is an important part of marketing to increase awareness of the product or service offered. Some examples of promotion include local radio or television news releases, direct mail pieces, paid advertisements in the local paper, or running a contest. The use of social media has become an important promotional activity that can help reach the target audience in a cost-effective manner. The price should be set after careful consideration of costs and what the marketplace will bear.

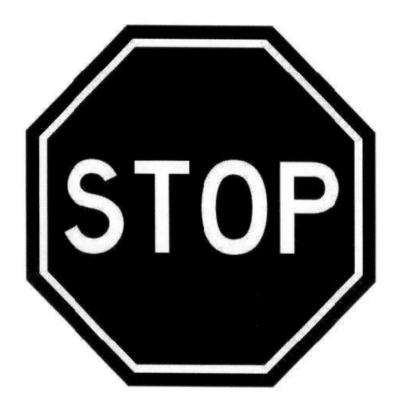

FREE Test Taking Tips DVD Offer

To help us better serve you, we have developed a Test Taking Tips DVD that we would like to give you for FREE. **This DVD covers world-class test taking tips that you can use to be even more successful when you are taking your test.**

All that we ask is that you email us your feedback about your study guide. Please let us know what you thought about it – whether that is good, bad or indifferent.

To get your **FREE Test Taking Tips DVD**, email freedvd@studyguideteam.com with "FREE DVD" in the subject line and the following information in the body of the email:

   a. The title of your study guide.

   b. Your product rating on a scale of 1-5, with 5 being the highest rating.

   c. Your feedback about the study guide. What did you think of it?

   d. Your full name and shipping address to send your free DVD.

If you have any questions or concerns, please don't hesitate to contact us at freedvd@studyguideteam.com.

Thanks again!

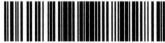

63316131R00110

Made in the USA
Middletown, DE
31 January 2018